THE
CAUSE
OF DEATH

Message from the author, Cynric Temple-Camp

ROYALTIES FROM THE SALE OF THIS BOOK

My office overlooks the rescue helicopter landing pad at Palmerston North Hospital. I am lucky to be able to watch the crew lifting off in their awesome machine just metres from the window. I see them scramble on average once a day, on missions to help the distressed and those who are injured. Their missions are literally a matter of life and death. They deliver the living to the waiting medical services. The dead come to us. They have been involved in so many of the cases I have investigated, including several events in this book. We all owe them a debt for the unceasing vigil they keep and the help they bring in times of tragedy. It is fitting that these tales belonging to the dead stand as a tribute to the work of the rescue teams.

I have therefore pledged to give all royalties from the sale of this book to the Palmerston North Rescue Helicopter, an essential emergency service for the Manawatu-Whanganui region.

THE CAUSE OF DEATH

DR CYNRIC TEMPLE-CAMP

HarperCollins*Publishers*

HarperCollins*Publishers*
First published in 2017
by HarperCollins*Publishers* (New Zealand) Limited
Unit D1, 63 Apollo Drive, Rosedale, Auckland 0632, New Zealand
harpercollins.co.nz

Copyright © Cynric Temple-Camp 2017

Cynric Temple-Camp asserts the moral right to be identified as the author of this work. This work is copyright. All rights reserved. No part of this publication may be reproduced, copied, scanned, stored in a retrieval system, recorded, or transmitted, in any form or by any means, without the prior written permission of the publisher.

HarperCollins*Publishers*
Unit D1, 63 Apollo Drive, Rosedale, Auckland 0632, New Zealand
Level 13, 201 Elizabeth Street, Sydney NSW 2000, Australia
A 53, Sector 57, Noida, UP, India
1 London Bridge Street, London, SE1 9GF, United Kingdom
2 Bloor Street East, 20th floor, Toronto, Ontario M4W 1A8, Canada
195 Broadway, New York NY 10007, USA

A catalogue record for this book is available from
the National Library of New Zealand

ISBN 978 1 7755 4109 7 (pbk)
ISBN 978 1 775 49140 8 (ebook)

Cover design by Darren Holt, HarperCollins Design Studio
Cover images: Road by Jill Ferry/Getty Images; scalpel by shutterstock.com
Typeset in Bembo Std by Kirby Jones
Printed and bound in Australia by McPhersons Printing Group
The papers used by HarperCollins in the manufacture of this book are a natural, recyclable product made from wood grown in sustainable plantation forests. The fibre source and manufacturing processes meet recognised international environmental standards, and carry certification.

CONTENTS

	Prologue	1
Chapter 1	The Makings of a Pathologist	7
Chapter 2	The Exhumation	32
Chapter 3	The Naked Woman	52
Chapter 4	A Tale of Two Publicans	63
Chapter 5	A Touch of Madness	87
Chapter 6	Drug Mule	109
Chapter 7	The Devil Comes to Town	118
Chapter 8	In the Arms of Ecstasy	132
Chapter 9	The Eggshell Skull	142
Chapter 10	Trouble with the Babysitter	169
Chapter 11	The Circumstances of Death	185
Chapter 12	The Smallest Speck of Evidence	199
Chapter 13	Accidents, Accidents, Accidents	219
Chapter 14	Questionable Evidence?	240
Chapter 15	Victims of a Disaster	249
Chapter 16	Dangerous Elements	272
Chapter 17	The Privy Council and Beyond	287
	Afterword	309

Prologue

The dead baby is gone, returned to her parents, but her presence lingers in the building. Questions have arisen from her death that remain like an unquiet spirit.

She presented as just another 'cot death', or SUDI (Sudden Death in Infancy) case. That, on my advice, was the Coroner's preliminary finding. Her little corpse was flawless, both externally and internally. If it weren't for the bluish pallor that had replaced the glow of vitality on her alabaster skin, she would have been the very picture of a healthy, well-cared-for little girl, plump and perfectly formed.

I had performed the usual array of tests. I had X-rayed her and examined the films minutely, looking for any evidence of the multiple rib and other fractures, old and new, that are known to indicate abuse, or what was once called 'Battered Baby Syndrome'. But the films were pristine, as I knew they would be. It's never quite that easy.

The Cause of Death

Next, there was an array of more invasive tests: careful and difficult dissections, using small scissors and scalpels specially designed for the task, for the purpose of collecting samples for detailed examination. I took spinal fluid by doing a lumbar puncture. This was negative for meningitis, or indications of any of the other, rarer diseases that can affect the brain and nervous system and cause sudden illness and death. I took swabs from the lungs, the throat, and the spleen, but there was no indication the infant had been carried off by an overwhelming bacterial infection such as by *Haemophilus influenzae*, which can cause rapid swelling of the larynx and a death by suffocation that is nearly as fast as meningitis.

I collected blood and tissue for the lab to look for a rare condition called QT syndrome. I had encountered this before, but it wasn't the cause of this little girl's death. I inserted a needle into the baby's sightless eyeball to extract fluid so that her electrolyte levels could be measured, but there were no abnormalities in the balance of sodium and potassium. And of course, I had taken tissue biopsies from every organ, fixed them on slides and, later, examined them under the microscope.

There was nothing out of the ordinary whatsoever.

It bothers me that she had died while being looked after by the babysitter. But I have come to the end of the set of investigations that the autopsy comprises, and I am no closer to determining a cause of death. It bothers me, but it won't be the first unresolved mystery I've had in my time and it certainly won't be the last.

Prologue

And now like an awful slow-moving dream, two years later it was all happening again to the same family: to her sister. Her paediatrician had visited me to discuss the case. 'Her sister died of cot death two years ago,' he said.

'I remember,' I said. 'I did the autopsy then.'

'So you remember she was with a babysitter the night she died. I told the family they should think carefully before they ever left their little one with that sitter again. The babysitter was a family friend and they supported her. But guess who was looking after her the night the second child died?'

I stared at him.

'That's got to be coincidence, doesn't it?'

'Well, I'm not so sure. Because over the last few months, they've brought her in several times for apnoeic attacks.'

'Interesting, but ...'

'And guess who was looking after her every time she stopped breathing in her sleep.'

'The babysitter? Really?'

He nodded.

The phone rings. It's my colleague, Dr Bruce Lockett, who is leading the investigation this time.

'Cynric, you won't believe this,' he says.

I listen as he tells me what has happened, and what he has found.

'What do you think it means?' I ask.

He isn't sure.

'Who can tell us what this means?' I think aloud.

'If anyone can, it would be David Becroft in Auckland,' says Bruce.

Both of us know that this is a step forward. I already feel a slight tingle of anticipatory excitement. We might get a resolution, after all.

Because, in the end, that's what the whole science of pathology is based upon: the belief that every death is a question that deserves — that demands — an answer.

* * *

Some of the stories in this collection have been reported elsewhere. Others are untold stories, relating my part in the unexpected deaths and accidents that have befallen others. I believe the stories of the dead should be told, as quite apart from anything else, they are our story, too. For as much as we don't like to talk about it or even to admit it to ourselves, death is our common destiny.

What's more, the living can learn much from the deaths of others. That is the whole point of pathology (literally, the study of death). From an analysis I once did on the many autopsies I have performed on people who have died in hospital, I have determined that only 40 per cent of patients die with the benefit of a correct diagnosis. In another 30 per cent, the right organ system is targeted, but the precise diagnosis has been wrong. For the remaining 30 per cent of patients, the diagnosis has failed to identify the correct organ, let alone the nature of the disorder. My findings are consistent with similar studies everywhere, even emanating from such an august body as America's prestigious Mayo Clinic.

Prologue

We do not need to be unduly alarmed by this, but nor should we shrug and cease to strive to do better, on the grounds that we are human and humans make mistakes. The science of pathology is dedicated to learning from human error.

There are indeed tales of woe here. Of course there are. For that is death, and that is life: happiness and woe.

CHAPTER 1

The Makings of a Pathologist

I had my first, up-close experience with death when I was growing up in the African nation that used to be known as Rhodesia. Like all white Rhodesian families, we had servants back then. Our cook Robert, his wife Samma, his daughter Tombi and his newborn son Samuel lived in a small brick and mortar outbuilding called a *kia*. Tombi was the same age as me and we were inseparable companions.

One morning when I was eight years old, my mother stopped me as I made to head over to the *kia* to play with Tombi as usual.

'Samuel has died,' she told me. 'The police are on their way.'

I wasn't entirely sure what she meant, and it made me more determined than ever to visit Tombi to find out what was happening. I managed to hold off until my parents retired for their post-lunch siesta, when I ran up the path to the *kia* to see for myself.

I found Robert outside, feeding blankets and clothing into a fire. I recognised the tiny items belonging to his son.

Robert glanced up at me as I ran up breathlessly and nodded at me solemnly.

'Robert, why are you burning your blankets?' I asked.

He looked at me again, and held my eye. I saw all the ancient anguish of Africa in that look, but I was too young to fully understand. A tear welled up in his eye. He dashed it away.

'It is because of what the witches have done that I must burn everything,' he replied.

I shivered despite the hot sun.

Later, I secretly went back to the site of the fire. Robert had buried all the burnt embers.

I dug them up, examining ash and fragments of clothes and blankets.

I have no idea why I did this. I was only eight years old. Perhaps I was looking for some traces of the witches. Or perhaps I was just curious and behaving like a nosey boy.

* * *

Years later I came across a different experience of death that had a significant similarity.

A prominent surgeon in the Cape went to play golf one afternoon with a few of his colleagues. He took his 13-year-old son to act as a caddy. Somewhere along the course the lad dropped dead before their eyes.

The Makings of a Pathologist

They did everything to resuscitate the boy, but to no avail.

The initial autopsy showed nothing, but the father could not accept that there could be no reason for his son's death. He wanted an answer. Day after day he harried the pathologists for progress. The cardiac pathology specialist, Dr Alan Rose, eventually dissected the conducting system of the boy's heart into hundreds of microscopic slides. Finally an answer: Alan found an abnormal conduction pathway that would have misdirected the electrical current and caused a ventricular fibrillation and sudden death.

Only then was the father prepared to let it go.

How are these stories similar?

All humans react in the same way to the unexpected death of their loved ones. It doesn't matter whether you are an African tribesman in the 1960s, or an orthopaedic surgeon in the 1980s, you will feel the death of your son similarly and keenly. And you will search until you have an explanation of why this tragedy has occurred.

Whether the answer that satisfies you lies in your certainty that we are afflicted by the dark forces of witchcraft, or whether you take comfort from the modern shamans — contemporary pathologists — the power of the explanation is the same. Nothing haunts as tenaciously as questions. Answers are like an exorcism, of sorts.

* * *

I emerged from my medical training with no clear idea about which branch of specialist medicine to pursue. But like most doctors, I began my career imagining I would be looking after the living rather than the dead. I graduated first from the University of Rhodesia and then from the Royal College of Surgeons of Edinburgh, shivering through the winter of my final exams in the Royal Infirmary.

After you had qualified and prior to registration, Rhodesian doctors were required to do a year in a hospital as a house surgeon, working you hard in medicine, general and neurosurgery. No sooner had I finished, I was called up for military service. The prospect was both daunting and exciting. Rhodesia had been in the grip of a brutal civil war since the early 1960s, and it was showing no signs of abating. I was assigned as an Air Force medical officer, and for 18 months I looked after the wounded from both sides and saw many who were beyond help. There was no sense or logic to the conflict as seen from the inside. There were just spells of intense boredom and sudden bursts of activity and fear. Mostly there was only a short, daily sick parade (soldiers' clinic) to occupy me; my medical orderly could have done this parade at least as competently as I could. Once the clinic was over, we read and waited and played bridge and waited again. A cup of tea or the next meal was about as exciting as it got.

Every so often, we would receive a call to perform a 'casevac', or casualty evacuation. Then, high with adrenaline and excitement, I would clamber into an Alouette III helicopter and we would thunder off to pick up injured soldiers or civilians. The civilians were usually victims of landmines, and the soldiers were generally casualties of bush contact with the insurgents. All too often, civilian or solider, they were dead when we arrived.

It was a hot October month when I was assigned to a Forward Airfield on the banks of the Zambesi River at Kariba. The daily sick parade was over and everything was coagulating into the accustomed boredom. I asked the Squadron Leader, our base commander, whether I could head up the hill to the local public hospital at Kariba to see if I could help out. The hospital was a simple, 25-bed facility with one operating theatre and an ancient X-ray machine. But with a catchment of 300,000 people living in the vicinity of Lake Kariba and the Zambesi valley, the hospital was always busy and the beds full. At least there, there would be something to do, and if I was needed on a casevac, the hospital was only three minutes from the base by helicopter. The Squadron Leader agreed on condition I undertook to be back within 20 minutes if something came up at base.

I took a Land Rover and headed into Kariba township. The District Medical Officer who was running the hospital, Diederik van der Byl, had been a senior surgical registrar when I did my stint as a house surgeon. Diederick was palpably relieved to see me, because as it turned out, there was a lot going on and in the middle of it all, he was facing the prospect of performing a double amputation.

I was quite well accustomed to the procedures for double amputations, as all too many victims of landmines suffered horrific injuries to both legs. This time, it was different. The patient was a German tourist, which was strange enough in this war-torn region. But what made it truly bizarre was that his injuries had been inflicted by a charging elephant. Upon spotting a herd close to the road, the man had stopped his car and got out to take a photograph. Thinking it would be better from a photographic perspective if the animals were flapping their ears, he began throwing stones at them. This had the desired effect, but after flapping its ears as a warning, one of the elephants charged. It was a miracle the animal didn't kill him outright.

I went up to the ward to see his injuries for myself. He was quite a sight. Two units of blood were running into him and there were tourniquets around his thighs, but he was pale as alabaster. There was a pulpy mush below his knees where his lower legs had been.

'The wife is hysterical,' Diederik told me. 'She's been on the phone to the German ambassador in Pretoria, telling him to fly in a planeload of specialists to save his legs. She's refusing to agree to the amputation.'

'What are you going to do?' I asked.

'I'm going ahead,' he shrugged. 'He won't make it otherwise. As soon as we can get him stable, we'll get him into theatre. Do you think you could give them a hand in maternity?'

In the maternity ward, I found five women in various stages of labour. I examined each of the women, checking their progress. Obstructed labour was common here, as the women of the valley were usually malnourished and had small pelvises. Intervention was required in about one in every four deliveries.

Sure enough, one woman was plainly in trouble. She had been 18 hours in labour, yet the head was still only three-fifths engaged and cervical dilation was dropping towards the minimum allowed. The birth process was in danger of stalling.

I listened through the ancient, tin ear-trumpet and found the foetal heart still okay. That was something.

I put up an oxytocin drip, and as the drug sped the contractions up, the cervix dilated. The head descended, but only as far as the pelvis, where it stuck. Now things started to go wrong. I listened, and found the beat regular at 130 beats per minute but dipping during the contractions. That deceleration of the baby's heartbeat was the first sign of foetal distress.

Quickly I injected the woman's perineum with local anaesthetic. I held out my hand and the midwife passed me a pair of scissors. I inserted two fingers between the stretched skin of the perineum and the baby's head and waited. As the next contraction bore down I slid one blade of the scissors between my fingers and snipped. Blood gushed over my hand as the skin split and the introitus gaped open.

'Let's have the ventouse,' I told the midwife assisting. She handed me the vacuum cup with its two handgrips. This suctions onto the baby's scalp and gives you purchase, providing you with a simple and relatively safe way to assist a slow second phase of birth.

While I awaited the next contraction, I placed the ear-trumpet to the woman's belly and listened to the baby's heart. It was down to 100 beats per minute now.

'We need this baby out fast,' I told the others in the room.

At this critical point, the Matron arrived and stood behind me.

'Doctor, you are wanted at the airfield,' she said.

My shoulders sagged. That gave me 20 minutes, but I needed 40 minutes at least to finish this delivery and get back.

The surge of the contraction began and I dragged steadily on the handles. The head began its descent, but the contraction was over too soon.

I listened to the baby's heart again: 96 beats per minute now.

If one more pull with the ventouse failed to bring the baby into the world, the options were diminishing. Normally, a Caesarean section would be performed, but Diederik's double amputation would have the operating theatre tied up for at least a couple of hours yet.

'Sister, can you get the Wrigley's forceps ready, please?' I asked. I didn't dare use the Kielland forceps. These are more efficient, but because they can reach higher in the maternal pelvis, you need to be experienced to use them safely.

All the while, I was trying not to imagine what the hell was happening at the airfield.

The next contraction came and I pulled as firmly and steadily as I dared.

'Push!' I implored the woman. 'Please push! This is important!'

She gave it everything, and the baby came!

I guided the head and pulled as the baby emerged, slowly at first, and then rapidly once the shoulders were clear. A boy. He gasped and began to wail. I handed the baby to the midwife and turned to tie off and cut the cord. I began to pull gently on the cord to deliver the placenta.

The baby was crying furiously. That was always the best sign, and I was beginning to allow myself to feel a sense of satisfaction. The placenta was delivered and it was intact and normal. Good. The midwife injected the baby with vitamin K to prevent neonatal bleeding and then prepared to inject the mother with Pitocin to prevent post-partum haemorrhage.

She looked strangely sombre. I looked at her enquiringly. She shook her head slightly, not making eye contact.

She passed me the baby. I looked and saw nothing. I turned the baby over.

A bulbous, membrane-bound nodule of tissue, known as a meningomyelocoele, protruded from the lower spine. My heart sank.

It was a spinal defect exposing the lower cord to the air — effectively a death sentence in tropical Africa, where disease is everywhere. There was nothing to be said or done that could make one shred of difference.

I turned back to my patient, my relief and sense of accomplishment snuffed and replaced by darkness. Methodically, I stitched the layers of her episiotomy closed. She lay still, her lips moving as she whispered something. As I tied the last suture off, I leaned forward to listen.

'Thank you, Doctor,' she breathed.

I realised, at that moment, I wasn't cut out for clinical medicine.

* * *

The Cause of Death

A helicopter clattered overhead, rattling the frame of the hospital building, and there was a whine as it altered pitch for landing. I pulled off my gloves, picked up my medical pack and ran outside. The machine was squatting on the pad, dust whirling in the wash from its blades. The technician gunner beckoned me and I ran, doubled over, beneath the blades. I pushed my medical kit aboard and clambered up after it, slipping past the twin Browning .303 machine guns. Once seated, I put on a headset and listened to the jumble of voices in the static.

'... hit a mine,' I heard. 'We're getting that it was a boosted mine. Total wreck and mass casualties. Many dead. We have one confirmed wounded, condition described as critical. Over.'

'Can you confirm location of LZ [landing zone]?' our pilot asked.

The reply placed the scene of the tragedy about 150 kilometres to our west towards Kanyemba.

We flew over African bush, brown and sere because the rains had not yet come. No trace of human life was visible, and the landscape looked as it had looked long before human beings first strode the plains of Africa. As I looked down out of the open door of the helicopter, I saw two adult elephants and their calf break away into the clear from where they had been browsing. In a flash we were past. Craning to see behind us, I saw their dark forms lumbering away, ears flapping.

There was a confusion of urgent voices in the earpieces of my headset. I couldn't quite follow what they were saying, but I thought I heard something about an aeroplane crash.

The Makings of a Pathologist

And sure enough, as a pall of smoke became visible rising from the bush ahead of us, I heard an anguished voice reporting that a plane was down at our destination.

When we landed, we learned that a light, single-engined Police Reserve Air Wing Cessna had landed on this bush strip to unload a four-man patrol of Game Park Rangers and had hit a boosted landmine cunningly planted by the insurgents. There were already three dead men and two more, despite my best efforts, soon would be from their horrific blast injuries.

The wreckage and bodies were spread over a large area. I stayed and helped with the retrieval. It was a harrowing, gory and gut-churning experience for a young doctor.

Once it was complete, I flew with the body bags containing the remains of the three victims back to Salisbury. After a haunted night, I presented myself to the mortuary the following morning to brief the pathologist on the circumstances. I was pleased to find it was Kevin Lee, the charismatic and entertaining forensic pathologist who had lectured us as medical students. I was supposed to leave the dead in his capable hands and return to Kariba as soon as possible, but at Kevin's invitation, I stayed to watch him at work. Kevin was instrumental in fostering my interest in pathology as a career.

Back in 1974, when I was a medical student, he had provided me with a brilliant demonstration of what is involved in investigating an air accident. That disaster back then involved a single-engined Aeromacchi A-60 Trojan that had loaded up a paramedic and a wounded man from a mined truck, with a view to flying them to assistance. But on lifting off from the rough, bush strip, the nose wheel of the plane had failed to clear a Land Rover parked at the end. After clipping it, the plane had pitched into the mopani trees and unforgiving ground beyond the strip at 80 knots, plenty fast enough to spread wreckage over a considerable area — and the bodies, of course.

Kevin taught me that it wasn't simply a matter of sweeping bodies into bags, as I had imagined. Instead, as I watched and listened, fascinated, he performed a careful dissection of the body parts, hunting for specific clues from which a narrative of the crash could be assembled.

Despite the terrible state of the bodies, he found them, too.

He dissected the pilot first, showing me how to distinguish the massive, deadly injuries inflicted by the impact from the subtle, specific ones that indicated his position relative to the controls. The left hand was a bag of crushed bones where the impact with the ground had been transmitted through the control column directly to the hand grasping it. Kevin explained that this indicated the pilot was conscious and manipulating the controls at the time. The right hand was lacerated and abraded but not fractured. This was also as expected, if the pilot were actively attempting to control the aircraft. His right hand would have been on the throttle.

Similarly, the pilot's right leg had been shattered by a blow of considerable force delivered to the underside of the heel. This was evidence that his foot was pushing on the right rudder bar at the instant of impact. Kevin deduced from this that the Trojan had yawed after clipping the Land Rover, dropping its wing to the left. The correct recovery response would be for the pilot to push the right rudder hard to the floor.

'We can safely say he was flying the thing,' Kevin said. 'He hadn't lost consciousness or been taken out by a sniper, or anything like that.'

The next subject for his investigations was the casualty whom the pilot was evacuating. Kevin found ample evidence that he had sustained a ruptured spleen and liver and was all but bled-out before the crash.

'He would have died of these injuries before he could reach help,' Kevin observed. 'No need for anyone else to have died on his behalf. Shame, really.'

* * *

Nearly four months after this incident, I was carrying out my afternoon surgery at the New Sarum Air Force Base for the wives and children of the serving men. I was peering down the ear canal of a nine-year-old with earache, at a red and infected eardrum.

I sighed.

I explained to the patient's mother that it was probably viral, and apart from prescribing a decongestant and a mild pain killer, there wasn't much I could do. It would clear up in its own good time.

'So you'll be giving him antibiotics, then, won't you,' she said.

The Cause of Death

I bit my tongue. Antibiotics wouldn't achieve anything, but I had been in this job long enough to know that any attempted explanation would achieve even less.

As I finished writing out the scrip, the practice nurse came in.

'The Base Commander would like to see you, Doctor,' she said.

My patient and his mother left as the New Sarum Base Commander came in, accompanied by Flight Sergeant Mills. I stood up, my bewilderment no doubt visible on my face. Flight Sergeant Mills was from security.

'Sorry to interrupt, Doctor,' the Base Commander said. My apprehension eased somewhat. Our rule of thumb in the medical corps was that being called 'Doctor' by senior officers was good. 'Doc' was even better. But if your rank was used, watch out!

The Commander sat down. Sergeant Mills remained standing at the door, somewhere between at attention and at ease.

'We understand you have human remains in your office,' the Commander said.

I nodded. A while before, another student had offered to sell me a wooden box containing a skull and half a skeleton. Its origins were unknown, but the remains were probably those of a pre-colonial tribesman. I bought it, and several of us had been using it for our anatomy studies. Pilots occasionally came in and asked to have a look: most people have a macabre interest in death. This was the 1970s and sensibilities were a far cry from what they are today, where we are conditioned to treat all human remains with respect. I thought nothing of keeping the bones, and was happy to show them off.

I opened the cupboard and placed the box on my desk. The Commander opened it and gazed inside. The empty eyesockets of the skull stared back at him.

'What the hell do you think you're doing, storing human remains in your office like they're some sort of souvenir? Have you got any idea how offensive that is, Flight Lieutenant?'

There it was. My rank.

'It's disgusting and disrespectful and downright immoral. What have you got to say for yourself?'

'Well,' I stammered. 'I had them as a sort of study aid. Several of us …'

'A study aid?' the Commander looked aghast. 'These are human remains, Flight Lieutenant! This is a dead person! Did you think to tell the principal Medical Officer that you were keeping a dead body in your office as a "study aid"?'

I shook my head.

'No, sir,' I mumbled.

The Commander stood up abruptly. So did I.

'You will make arrangements for this,' he gestured at the box, 'to be given a decent burial forthwith. Sergeant Mills will take charge of it. Carry on.'

He left. After the door banged shut, I turned bleakly to Flight Sergeant Mills. His shoulders were shaking with laughter.

'Should have seen your face!' he wheezed. 'What a bollocking!'

I found myself beginning to smile and then to laugh, too. Soon we were both laughing uproariously. As I laughed, I felt a bit better, but I was certain of one thing. I was no more cut out for military life than I was for clinical medicine. I still had years of military service in prospect. I wondered how I would stand it.

* * *

And then, suddenly, soon after that incident, that part of my life was over. The war ended. We had lost. Robert Mugabe had won. Within a week, I was discharged from the Air Force. I was penniless, but I was back with my wife, Elayne, and free again to choose my path in life and in medicine.

But what to do? Thoughts of pursuing pathology had visited me from time to time while I was a student. I'd always enjoyed anatomy and dissection and had excelled at histology, the examination of tissue under the microscope. And now Elayne reminded me of how fascinated I had been by the air crash autopsies. Perhaps I should give pathology a go, and see whether I could make a life for myself amongst the dead.

Two days later we arrived in Cape Town, the sea beneath dashing itself against a savage coast as the plane trembled and lurched in the high wind. It was all very different — wild, cold and beautiful — compared to the high and hot savannah where I grew up.

I had an appointment to see Professor Dirk Uys, head of pathology at the world-renowned Groote Schuur Hospital.

The Makings of a Pathologist

I was shown into his office, the walls of which were lined with books. I learned later that Professor Uys had a copy of just about everything ever written on the subject of pathology, right back to *Patologie Anschrift,* written by Rudolph Virchow, the so-called father of pathology, first published over a century ago.

Professor Uys himself was regarding me over his huge desk. He was internationally famous for his original work on the very first case of heart transplant and was an expert in mesotheliomas, the malignant tumours afflicting the linings of the lung that are caused by blue asbestos.

He motioned me to the chair in front of his desk. It was small, hard, wooden, and upright. I would come to know that chair well.

When I told him the purpose of my visit — that I would like to become a pathologist and was seeking his advice — he grimaced and shook his head.

'Do you know how difficult it is to get a position as a pathology registrar, young man? There are dozens of applicants every year. And it doesn't help that you have presented yourself now. The academic year begins in January, and here we are in July.'

I told him that my sudden discharge from the Rhodesian Air Force had left me unemployed.

'I will see what can be done,' he said, noncommittally.

I left his office, feeling much discouraged. But only a matter of a few days later, Professor Uys called to say that one of the current intake of registrars had resigned, as he felt general practice would suit him better.

'So we have a vacant position,' Professor Uys said. 'Of course, you are some months behind and will have to work very hard to catch up. Would you accept it, if we make the offer of a place?'

'You bet I would,' I said, and just like that, I was enrolled, without even having to undergo the difficult and highly competitive selection process held every November. Perhaps pathology was meant to be.

* * *

Everything else I had done — my medical training, my exams in Edinburgh — all seemed easy compared with the demands of every day of the five years of my pathology training. For 12 hours a day, every day, I read textbooks and journals, studied tens of thousands of glass slides under the microscope, dissected organs and, of course, assisted with or performed hundreds of autopsies.

At first, I found the autopsies ghastly. Not only was there the cold, unnatural stiffness of the refrigerated dead, but also the strange, cloying smell of decay that seemed to persist long afterwards, despite the two pairs of gloves I wore while at work and the endless scrubbing I did after pulling them off. But gradually, I became accustomed to these aspects, and became more and more engaged with the detective work that is involved. As I honed my skills, I started discovering things, noticing things — small things at first, but with time and experience, I developed the ability to fit my observations into bigger and more complete puzzles.

The Makings of a Pathologist

Every Friday lunchtime, there was an autopsy meeting in the lecture hall in the mortuary. The pathology consultants would all gather around a presentation table laden with that week's supply of body parts, while the medical and surgical consultants sat in the surrounding amphitheatre to hear the exegesis of their patients' organs and learn what they had missed. It was fascinating and frightening time for the registrars: Professor Uys stood in the centre pointing out pathology of interest with a small retractable pointer and barking question at us. He was scathing if you didn't have the answers.

These days, we replace all organs. That is, everything that is removed for dissection — hearts, lungs, brains, everything relevant to disease — is put back in the body and the body closed up before being released to the family for the funeral. Back in the 1980s, the body cavities were stuffed with sawdust, while the organs were pickled in formalin and saved up for presentation at the weekly meeting. Sometimes, when it had been necessary to remove the spine, the body was braced with a broomstick and closed and released.

After the meeting, Sam, the Zulu mortuary assistant, would collect all the pickled organs into a bag and have them incinerated — at least, in theory. One of the distractions from my studies came when we learned that Sam had been caught selling organs to a witchdoctor to make traditional tribal medicine. I had heard similar stories in Rhodesia. One of the government medical officers in Gwelo (now Gweru) had told me about a body that had been discovered by the side of the road, apparently the victim of a hit-and-run. The police soon determined he had been run over by a truck and as there were only a few trucks on that road that night, they were soon able to find the driver. When interviewed, he said the body was already dead, and that this was an old trick: when the driver stopped to check on the person he had struck, a gang of bandits would come out and rob him. The police took the body along to the government mortuary where it was confirmed there were major injuries consistent with it having being run over by a truck. But strikingly, the brain was missing. It had been rather crudely removed, and it was eventually determined that the body had been illegally acquired from a hospital mortuary and the brain removed by one of the local witchdoctors. The witchdoctor couldn't be found, as he had already absconded into the bush.

We all thought Sam would be arrested and imprisoned, which we were sorry about — we all liked him and he was very good at his job — but something must have been worked out on the quiet. He reappeared in our midst, much chastened and determined not to get involved in this grisly trade again.

That was one interesting interlude. Another came when one day Professor Uys asked me to demonstrate an autopsy to an artist, a simply dressed, 20-something woman with solemn eyes and middle-parted light brown hair. She explained that she thought she would be able to capture her human subjects better from the outside if she knew what they looked like on the inside.

'Do you know much about anatomy?' I asked her as we prepared.

The Makings of a Pathologist

'Nothing,' she said, eyeing the greyish body nervously. 'I don't even know where poos are kept.'

It seems strange to me now that she was allowed to observe, but everything was more casual in those days. To the uninitiated, autopsies are the stuff of nightmares, really. The young woman was quiet throughout, and watched intently. She later sent me a drawing of the experience and her feelings while watching me carry out the autopsy. It is a striking picture and we keep it framed on the wall of our bedroom.

* * *

Professor Uys had told me at the beginning of my training that I was required to know the pathology of every disease of every organ of the body. More than that, I would have to be familiar with the clinical presentation of each of these diseases as well as have an idea of how they should be treated. There was nothing that might not be relevant to pathology, except psychiatry — and even that could be important, on occasion.

The first test of my aptitude came when a morbidly obese man died suddenly on the wards one weekend. I performed the autopsy and was able to diagnose a ruptured aortic aneurism as the cause of death. I did a careful dissection showing all of the pathology and was able to answer every question thrown at me. Professor Uys nodded approvingly at me before the group moved on to the next complicated case.

The next and by far the more gruelling test was the final examinations. Pass, and I would qualify as a specialist pathologist. Fail and, well, that would be four wasted years.

More than half those who sat the exams in any given year would fail.

There were two three-hour exam papers, six essays per paper, and as Professor Uys had indicated, it seemed they covered every disease of every organ in every imaginable particular. The questions were diabolical.

'Describe the findings at autopsy in a 22-year-old African male who has died as a result of Keto-acidotic coma from diabetes.'

The answer was simple, surely? Death would be metabolic, due to electrolyte and blood-sugar imbalances. This would leave no trace that could be seen in an autopsy. Of course, one could collect fluid from the eyeball, to demonstrate the potassium and glucose levels, but there would be nothing else to find. The answer — 'Nothing' — took no more than two minutes to arrive at and write.

A wave of doubt washed over me. Why had they allotted 30 minutes for a two-minute answer? What was I missing? But I reassured myself that the answer had to be right, and forced myself to move on.

After the three days that the written part of the exam occupied, it was time for the dreaded practical. Twenty glass slides of difficult and exotic diseases, each accompanied with a short clinical history, were presented for me to examine under the microscope. My task: make 20 diagnoses and supply appropriate clinical recommendations, all in writing. No mistakes were permitted.

I found nothing to be particularly fazed about, and afterwards, as I paced up and down outside the examination hall, waiting to hear my fate, I was quietly confident. Eventually, the door opened.

'Will you come in, sir? The examiners are ready for you.'

I went through the heavy doors into the great hall. Two professors sat behind a desk: Professor Uys, of course, and Professor Weber from Stellenbosch University in the Boland. They looked at me and I searched their expressions for any indication of congratulation or commiseration. Their faces were impossible to read.

My heart sank. What did this mean? Had I failed?

'Doctor,' said Professor Weber, 'we have put a slide on the microscope in front of you. Please be good enough to examine it and give us your opinion.'

I had trouble working the focus wheels on the microscope with my trembling fingers, but eventually the stained features of the tissues on the slide sharpened into brilliant clarity.

Concentrate, I told myself. Start at the beginning. Get a history before making a diagnosis: that's what Professor Uys always says.

I looked up, cleared my throat and asked if there was any relevant history. My voice sounded wobbly, but Professor Weber nodded in approval.

'No,' he said. 'There is no relevant history.'

I looked down and re-examined the slide.

The cells I could see were a sample from an acute appendicitis, with peritonitis: that much was obvious. This was a very common diagnosis. Surely they wouldn't be giving me *this* as a final examination case? What was I missing?

The Cause of Death

Always get all the information, Prof Uys was in the habit of telling us. We are the detectives. We need to know everything. We need to discover everything. Don't miss any clue, no matter how trivial. Always look at the slide, check the name — look for any information that might be available.

I looked down at the slide and read the patient's name. Siganada Sekunza.

That sounded like a Zulu name to me. I felt my mind begin to work.

Acute appendicitis is common in the West, but very rare amongst Africans, except — now my mind was really working — in Zululand, where amoebic appendicitis was quite common.

I re-examined the slide, and now that I was looking, there they were: two amoebae, right on the corner of the slide, almost obscured by pus.

Elation welled up within me.

Keeping my expression professional and neutral, I looked up and met Professor Weber's eyes.

'Sir, this is a case of amoebic appendicitis.'

He nodded, and it was as though the sun had burst through the clouds. Suddenly, both professors were smiling at me. They stood up and congratulated me, shaking my hand and slapping me on the back.

It was over, I realised with a feeling of disbelief. I had passed. I was now a pathologist.

The examiners invited me to share a celebratory glass of dry Cape sherry and then I raced home to Elayne, who was pretending to be absorbed with the gardening. Having supported me through all the long days and sleepless nights these last five years, she had nearly as much invested as me.

'So, don't you want to know how I got on?' I said.

She shrugged, affecting nonchalance, and carried on weeding.

'I passed,' I said. 'Now we can get on with our lives.'

CHAPTER 2

The Exhumation

After a stint as a specialist on the staff of Groote Schuur Hospital, I was lucky enough to secure a position as a pathologist at Palmerston North Hospital in the Manawatu, in the lower North Island of New Zealand. After our arrival in New Zealand and negotiating a mountain of paperwork for various government departments in Wellington, Elayne, our baby son Richard and I set off to start our new life.

I was welcomed to Palmerston North Hospital by Mr David Chrisp, the Medical Superintendent, and Dr Roy Darby, the Head of Pathology, who showed me about the hospital — most notably the mortuary and the laboratory — and introduced me to some of the people with whom I would be working. Then he gave me a starched white coat, a pager and a brown badge embossed with my name and showed me to a small, windowless office with a desk and telephone.

'This is yours,' he said, and left me to it.

The Exhumation

No sooner had I sat down and cast a single, bleak glance around my office than the phone rang, startling me. It was so soon that I supposed it had to be a wrong number.

'Hello?' I said tentatively.

'Is that the pathologist?'

'Yes,' I replied. 'Dr Temple-Camp speaking.'

There was a short pause, while the caller processed my name and my accent.

'Who did you say?'

'Dr Temple-Camp. I'm the pathologist. Can I help you?'

'Temple-Camp? Oh, I see.'

The caller told me that he was a detective sergeant with the CIB, the Criminal Investigation Branch.

'Yes, Detective Sergeant,' I said. 'What can I do for you?'

'We need you to come for an exhumation.'

An exhumation! I had never done one before. I had seen many dead people, but I'd never yet had to dig one up out of the ground, and this was far from what I'd expected of my first day on the job in New Zealand.

'Why does the body need to be exhumed?' I asked, naively assuming you could get simple, concise answers out of your solid, provincial New Zealand policeman. In his own, laconic way and in his own time, the detective sergeant told me that the grave in question had apparently been interfered with in some undefined way, and we had to find out why and by whom.

I persisted, until I further gathered that an object that had been identified as the nameplate from the lid of a coffin had been found lying above ground in the Foxton graveyard.

The mystery the police were seeking to solve was how it had got there.

My heart sank even further. I wondered how decomposed the body would be. Oh God. My stomach gave a nauseous heave at the thought.

'I suppose we'll be doing this in the middle of the night by the light of flaming torches?' I said.

The policeman didn't laugh.

'Well, not exactly,' he said. 'We're going to get cracking at four in the morning. We don't want the kids walking past while we're doing it. The earliest we can expect them to start coming by is seven. And actually, we won't be using flaming torches.'

* * *

After I had put down the phone, I pulled out my stained and battered copy of *Knight's Forensic Pathology*. I read and re-read the chapter on exhumations. It was surprising what you could learn from a decomposed body if you looked hard enough. I studied the pictures. They were appalling pictures of liquid things, barely recognisable as bodies, but as I read on, I became more and more interested. Some amazing findings were possible, even after years of underground decomposition, if you were persistent and diligent enough.

That afternoon, as I packed overalls, gloves, aprons, test tubes — anything I thought might be useful — Bruce Scott, the chief mortuary assistant, was sharpening the knives, the wheel singing as he ground the edges, his lips pursed as he frowned at the rooster-tail of orange sparks. He stopped what he was doing, put down the knife he was working on and began rummaging in a wooden chest in the corner of the mortuary.

'Here you go,' he said, pulling out an ancient-looking gas mask. 'It used to belong to Dr Pullar. He wore it whenever he had a really decomposed body to autopsy.'

Thomas Pullar was one of my predecessors. I took the mask and examined it with interest. Here, surely, was a Great War veteran. The round eyepieces looked like the eyes of an insect, while the corrugated proboscis was cracked and the powdery residue of perished rubber sifted over my hands.

I tried it on. The eyepieces were too far apart and I could barely see the through the opaque and scratched lenses. I sniffed. The smell was of rubber, and something else.

'It smells like a decomposing corpse,' I said.

'Quite possible,' Bruce replied. 'Dr Pullar didn't hold with rubber gloves, and he never changed his clothes for his autopsies. He just pulled a rubber apron over his suit and got on with it.'

'Really?'

'Yep. And he often smoked his pipe while he was doing autopsies. They tell me that, before my time, they once found him with his sandwiches sitting on the table while he was cutting up a septic spleen.'

This is the kind of detail that would have impressed Bruce, because as I got to know him, I found that his own standards of hygiene bordered on the obsessive-compulsive. He spent every moment he could spare from his routine duties scrubbing, swabbing and polishing. It wasn't a bad tic for a mortuary assistant to have.

I hastily tugged at the mask to get it off. The nose finally gave up its tenuous hold on life and crumbled into pieces of rubber that pattered onto the spotless tiled floor. Bruce looked down at with an expression of mingled sorrow and reproach.

He picked up a broom and swept the detritus into a pile, scowling and shaking his head.

With no gas mask at my disposal, I packed some cloth surgical masks instead, hoping for the best. Bruce smirked, but said nothing. He was a very experienced assistant. He knew that an ordinary cloth mask would be of no use for what I had coming in the next morning.

In the evening, I went to bed early, hoping that I could put the night's work out of my mind sufficiently to get a bit of sleep before the alarm went off. Fat chance. As I lay there, listening to Elayne breathing softly and steadily beside me, I kept going pointlessly over and over my preparations. Every few minutes, I would lift my head to check the time. It seemed to be standing still.

* * *

The alarm shrilled. I had gone to sleep after all.

As I climbed out of bed, I looked enviously down at Elayne. She pulled the duvet up around her chin, rolled on her side and sighed contentedly. I dressed, putting on an extra parka against the biting cold, and 15 minutes later I was

The Exhumation

leaving the lights of Palmerston North behind and driving into the blackness of the countryside to the south. The roads were deserted. Nothing moved. I shivered, as much with the cold as with apprehension, because it had been many years since the heater in my car — a dilapidated old Toyota — had worked.

There was a flash of light mist in the headlights and all of a sudden, I was driving in dense fog. The headlights reflected back at me as though off a wall, and I had to squint against the glare. My jaw ached, and I realised my teeth were tightly clenched. I slowed to a crawl. It was all I could do to stay on the narrow, winding road.

Eventually I came to Foxton. It was a typical small New Zealand town with a straggle of buildings, a hotel — closed, of course — several shops, houses and a cenotaph. I drove along the main street and saw nobody. Everything was in darkness. I knew the cemetery couldn't be far. I turned up an unmarked side road and followed it into the mist. The tarseal ended abruptly and I found myself bumping along a rutted, corrugated track. As I rounded a corner, the road petered out into a rubbish dump.

I retraced my steps and tried the next turn. This looked better. The road veered left and then right and the car clattered over a small bridge. According to my dim recollection of the road map, this didn't seem right, either, but the road was so narrow that I couldn't turn around. I pressed on and when the opportunity to turn left presented itself, I took it. I reasoned that if the cemetery wasn't down here, at least I would end up on the main road again.

The Cause of Death

After several minutes of groping along the road in the fog, I realised I was completely lost. This was the first job I'd had in my new role. Not only was I going to be late but it looked as if I might not get there at all. I might even have to be rescued. My only hope was to keep driving to see if I could pick up the main road, or a perhaps a signpost. I wasn't optimistic.

There was a flash of movement on the right. I experienced a surge of renewed hope, but it was only a flock of sheep blundering away from the car. At least there was some life in this dense mist. I drove on.

Suddenly, a figure loomed out of the mist, waving authoritatively at me. Behind it, I could make out a police car parked across the road.

This must be it.

I wound down the window and greeted a policewoman who pointed into the mist beyond the car.

'Cemetery's that way,' she said. 'They're all waiting for you.'

Relieved, I got out, opened the boot, took out my suitcase of tools, my gumboots, a surgical gown and a rubber apron. I strode off in the direction she had indicated, but within seconds, the fog had closed in once more and it was as if my car, her car and the policewoman herself had never existed. Where was everyone?

Should have brought a torch, I reproached myself.

I shuffled along the verge until I reached a gate. The fog swirled and there was a flicker of light away to my left. Never has anyone been so grateful to arrive at a graveyard in the

The Exhumation

middle of a dark, foggy night! At least I was here and could begin. I felt more sanguine about the whole enterprise. I'm a trained pathologist, I reminded myself. I can do this. I just have to pretend I know what I'm doing.

Through the mist, and by the uncertain illumination of the light I was walking towards, I could make out the outline of gravestones. Beyond them, standing under the dripping foliage of a few disconsolate trees, were a number of dark figures holding torches. One of them coughed and moved towards me.

At first I thought his form was being amplified in silhouette, but as he grew more substantial, he did not diminish. He was solid, all right, and his handshake was like a vice.

'Gidday,' he said. 'We're right over here.'

He led me towards the dark figures assembled beneath the trees.

I was amazed at how many people there were: a senior policeman with gold on his cap — the District Commander, perhaps, or someone of similar high rank — half a dozen constables, three men from the local undertakers', a man from the Ministry of Health whose name I didn't catch and the Reverend Father Patrick from All Saints Cathedral with his surly-looking sexton.

The detective outlined the story. A member of the public visiting the cemetery had found a brass nameplate lying on the grass. To their horror, they saw that it corresponded with the name on the grave 15 metres away. The finder took the plate to the police station. The local constable examined the grave and thought there were signs it had been interfered with. The detective he called wasn't so sure. But he consulted the undertakers who had performed the deceased woman's funeral.

The undertaker stepped forward. He had driven the hearse to the cemetery ready to receive the body, and he was standing there incongruously in the torchlight in his professional attire of dark tailcoat and waistcoat and dove-grey cravat. Something about his manner told me there was no way in the world he was going to miss this drama. He confirmed that the plate engraved for the deceased on the 14th of last month and which he had personally screwed onto the coffin lid was the one found on the lawn. His colleague, just as sharply dressed, nodded in affirmation.

'What did she die from?' I asked.

The detective pulled out his notebook, licked his finger and began flipping awkwardly through the book with one hand as he held his torch with the other.

'Here we go,' he said. 'She died of ish … isk …'

He had several goes at pronouncing ischaemic cardiomyopathy. Coronary artery disease, I thought. Nothing unusual there. Most people died of that in the developed world.

She had even had an autopsy to prove it, carried out by the temporary pathologist who acted as locum while the hospital waited for me to arrive from Africa.

The deceased had been living with her husband of 34 years at the time of her death. No children. She had been unwell for some months and the only real surprise was that she had predeceased her husband, who was ailing more than she was. There were no peculiar circumstances, family disputes or

The Exhumation

strange religious cults involved. The death and burial had been ordinary in every way.

There was no clue in her history as to the strange turn of events.

The local constable had his say next.

'This is a quiet area with nothing much happening. A pretty law-abiding community, really. A bit of drinking after closing time in the bar, the odd drunk in charge of a vehicle, a bit of fighting now and then. That's about it. Never anything like this before.'

Everybody seemed to have their story to tell. I felt I needed to take control. After all, this was supposed to be a pathological investigation. What was I supposed to do? The man from the Ministry took an envelope from his pocket, stepped forward and handed me a paper. It was a warrant signed by the Minister of Health authorising the exhumation of the deceased.

What on earth was I expected to do with this?

I folded it and stuffed it into my trouser pocket. I looked grave. That seemed to be sufficient. I nodded and we began.

* * *

The sexton — a scrawny but wiry redhead of about 30 years of age, wearing overalls and black army boots — picked up a shovel, drew in a deep breath and moved to the edge of the grave. Struck by a thought, he put down the shovel, fumbled in his pack and drew out a gas mask, the twin of the one I had inadvertently destroyed. He put on the mask, adjusted and tightened the straps, picked up the shovel again and began digging.

After about a quarter of an hour, the sexton flung the spade to the ground and ripped off his gas mask. His hair was matted, his face was puce and, despite the chill, beaded with sweat. He was panting heavily.

'Too fucken hot in that thing!'

He threw the mask to the ground and looked up at Father Patrick.

'Pardon the language, Father.'

He dug in his pack again and pulled out a water bottle, gulped at it thirstily, screwed on the lid and began digging once more. We watched from the side. The pile of earth grew and grew but the hole never seemed to get any deeper.

It was some time before the sexton gave a low whistle. We crowded forward and looked down into the grave. There were several crushed and withered flowers and a ribbon. He reached down and passed them up. More fragments of flowers surfaced as he dug deeper. He was sweating freely and by now had undone the top part of his overalls, shrugged his arms and shoulders out and tied the arms around his waist. I could see his muscles straining as he panted, lifting heavy shovelful after shovelful of the dark earth up and out.

I became aware that I could dimly see the outlines of the gravestones around us. I glanced at my watch. A quarter to six. Dawn was coming.

The detective had clearly come to the same realisation.

'Come on, man. Faster,' he urged. 'The school kiddies will be along soon. We've got to be out of here by then.'

The Exhumation

The sexton stopped, leaned on his shovel and fixed the detective in a baleful glare.

'It's pretty fucken hard going, mate, let me fucken tell you,' he said. 'If you think you can fucken do better, then don't let me stop you. Fill your boots.'

I was mildly shocked at the time, but I would soon come to realise that this was a pretty average provincial New Zealand conversation.

I felt sorry for the sexton. Still, soon his job would be over and then it would be my turn to perform. I can't say I was looking forward to it.

At last the coffin was exposed. The sexton climbed out of the grave, hurled his shovel to the ground, and began pulling up his overalls. That was all he was going to do. He looked down at the coffin and spat to the side in a way that suggested that actually opening it was way above his pay grade.

The reluctant Foxton constable was ordered into the grave to get the lid off the coffin. I felt sorry for him, too, but was relieved it wasn't me down there. He took his helmet off, placed it carefully beneath a tree and lowered himself into the grave. His boots thudded on the dirt-encrusted wood. The wood was surprisingly glossy as he shone his torch up and down the lid. The beam stopped on the discoloured patch where the plate had been torn off.

It didn't look as though anyone had been further than that, and at the same moment the thought occurred to me, the police officer looked up hopefully. I wondered what the view was like: our faces lined up around the pit and looking down at him, like mourners.

The Cause of Death

'The lid's got to come off,' the detective said.

'Bloody oath,' muttered the sexton. 'After all that.'

The officer struggled, which was hardly surprising, given he was trying to lift the lid while standing on it. He had to brace his feet against the walls of the grave and try to lever up the lid without falling forward onto the coffin. He was a big man. Who knows what would have happened if he had.

'There's a bit of trick to getting the lid off,' the undertaker said, and proceeded to try to explain it. It was incomprehensible to me and of no more use to the policeman. There was nothing for it but for the undertaker to go down and help. The constable came out of the grave with surprising alacrity.

The undertaker took his place, knelt on the coffin lid and undid the clasps. Even having seen it done, I couldn't tell you how he did it, but without apparent effort, the lid suddenly flew up out of the hole and landed on the pile of soil that the sexton had so laboriously scooped out. It was followed at high speed by the undertaker.

A cloying miasma followed him and spread thickly over us. We all backed off. The sexton, who had put his mask back on in anticipation, vomited into it. He wheeled away, tearing it off his head as he ran into the darkness. There was a twang and a strangled curse as he fell heavily over a strand of wire.

The smell of fresh vomit mixed with the other, strange odour. The District Commander grabbed his nose, clapped a hand over his mouth, turned and staggered into the trees. The sound of retching soon reached us.

The Exhumation

The detective swung his head challengingly around the lower ranks. Although wavering, they clenched their jaws and stood their ground. I knew how they felt. I had only just managed to keep my heaving stomach under control. Everyone was looking at me. It was my turn. I could hear Father Patrick praying quietly in Latin. It sounded mystical in that misty dawn.

With a confidence I did not feel, I stepped to the edge of the grave and looked down. It was definitely much lighter now and I could see clearly.

I frowned, or perhaps I flinched. This wasn't what I expected at all.

There lay the shrouded body, glowing — really, luminously glowing — whiter than any white I'd ever seen before. And it was hard to focus on the shape, as though it was fuzzy, or even furry.

The detective was at my side, looking at me questioningly. I shook my head. It was plain the body was undisturbed. I knew I would have to go down to have a closer look, just to be sure. There was probably still a smell of death and decomposition, but I had stopped noticing it. Something very strange was happening. There was a distinctive tinge of something else, something sweet, rather like molasses or honey. I just couldn't place the smell.

I picked up the lid of the coffin and turned it over. I don't know what ghoulish impulse made me do it, but I wasn't alone in feeling it. Everyone crowded around and a torch played up and down its underside as we examined it for scratch marks. There was nothing there to see, of course.

The Cause of Death

I climbed carefully into the hole and balanced myself on the edges of the coffin. To fall now would be catastrophic. The sweet smell was almost overpowering down in the pit. I could see that it wasn't the shroud that we were looking at. Instead, the shrouded cadaver was covered in a fine, fibrous coat, like candyfloss. At once, I recognised the sweet smell: it was just like candyfloss.

I brushed it lightly with my finger. It felt slimy to my touch, but not unpleasant.

I realised that a fuzz of saprophytic fungus had grown over the shroud while lying six feet down in the darkness of the earth. It was as white as white could be, glowing with bioluminescence.

With arms folded across her chest, the gleaming white body seemed strangely peaceful. We were intruding. The living didn't belong here in the deep realm of the dead. I climbed out of the grave.

'No sign of any interference whatsoever,' I announced. 'I don't think we need to get the body out. She's had an autopsy, and nothing's happened since.'

Everyone visibly slumped in relief.

'Could there be another body buried underneath the coffin?' asked the senior policeman, who had rejoined us, wiping his mouth.

Everyone looked at him with distaste.

'Well, it would be the perfect place to bury a body, wouldn't it?' he said, spreading his hands defensively. 'Who would ever look underneath a body that had already been buried?'

The Exhumation

We all turned and looked back into the grave. The sense of tranquillity still emanated. Time was marching on. Children were stirring in their warm beds. School was calling. We all felt it.

The detective took over and shook his head. The coffin hadn't been moved. We — or, more accurately, the undertaker and the sexton — closed up. It was a quarter to seven as we were treading down the earth over the grave. We were just in time. The mist was clearing and school was calling.

When I got home an hour later, Elayne was making breakfast. Our golden labrador puppy circled and leapt from side to side, wildly wagging her body in welcome, her face grinning in delight. The delicious aroma of eggs and bacon wafted through the house. I sat down with a cup of coffee.

The sense of normality in our kitchen was so profound that I could hardly believe where I had been and what I'd just been doing. Life was great now that this ordeal was over, and the memories were sufficiently surreal that when Elayne slid a plate of bacon and eggs in front of me, I found I was ravenously hungry.

It was only after I'd enjoyed my breakfast that I began to feel a sense of disappointment. We still didn't know who had disturbed the grave, and why. And I had no idea what the sweet smell emanating from the body was.

* * *

When I carried all my equipment back into the mortuary, Bruce was making a show of being busy with the mopping.

The Cause of Death

'Hello, Bruce,' I said casually.

He grunted, but there was an air of expectancy. I busied myself with putting all my gear away and kept him hanging.

Finally, Bruce could bear it no more. He had been expecting a badly decomposed body to autopsy, but I had arrived empty-handed. I relented and told him she'd already been autopsied.

'Oh?' he said. 'What name?'

There was an excellent chance he'd know the details of the case, and sure enough, when I told him the woman's name, he rolled his eyes. He knew something.

Bruce told me the woman's husband had been phoning him almost every day and had even been into the mortuary several times. He was convinced that his wife had been buried alive, and was perhaps, even now, still alive. The poor man was sure he could hear her screaming at night as she struggled to get out.

Bruce did his best to convince him that she was dead, all right, as dead as anybody could be. Even if she hadn't been dead when she came down from the ward to the mortuary, then she sure as hell was dead after the autopsy was over. Even this didn't make any difference. The poor, deluded fellow became a pest and Bruce eventually had to put a stop to it by threatening to report him to the police if he didn't desist.

My mouth was open. This was astonishing. Obviously the husband was the culprit.

I phoned the detective and told him what I'd just heard. He didn't sound surprised, and said he'd look into it.

The Exhumation

It turned out that Bruce had the right answer. The deceased's husband had been quite convinced that his wife was still alive, and decided he had to dig her up and prove it. He too knew he'd have to have it done by dawn because of the kids passing on their way to school, so he arrived at midnight and began digging. The sexton had found it hard going, and he was a young man turning over soil that had already been dug over once. The husband was in his seventies and had a bad heart as well as trouble with his hips. Apparently he'd dug and dug, stopping every now and then when his chest pains became too much. He reached the coffin just as dawn was breaking. He was desperate. He tried to pull the coffin lid off, but had no more luck than the local constable. He didn't know how to work the catches.

He stood on the coffin lid pulling, swearing and heaving, but couldn't get it to budge. Eventually, the truth dawned on him. He knew what everyone else had been trying to tell him all this time. His wife really was dead and gone.

He was surprised to hear about the nameplate. He couldn't remember pulling it off.

Would he be charged? Was this really a crime as such? The technical answer was yes, but he was clearly a man tormented. The police are pragmatists and used their discretion. No harm had been done — except for the waste of our time, of course — but he obviously had problems. The detective explained to him that our examination of the body had proved beyond doubt that she was, and always had been, dead, but it made little difference. He was referred to his general practitioner, who sent him to a psychiatrist.

Later that night, I sat at the kitchen table with Elayne drinking a cup of tea, and telling her the strange outcome. We talked about the poor husband. What made this man think that his wife could possibly be alive underground? How did he keep up such beliefs in the face of overwhelming evidence? He was entirely normal in every other way, so far as anyone could tell. My first professional case had opened for me a new field that I came to think of as forensic psychopathy, and about which I knew absolutely nothing. I had trained for years in the pathology of injury, disease and death, but I had little idea about the thoughts, the passions and the personalities that motivated those same bodies in life. Why should I? It was not part of my training, but I decided I would have to learn about this fascinating subject.

Vivisepulture is the accidental burial of a live person, and taphophobia (the fear of being buried alive) is said to be quite common. Elaborate 'safety' coffins with systems of rope, pulleys and a warning bell were popular in the 1800s. I wondered if this poor chap suffered from this phobia and somehow transferred his delusion to his interred wife.

And what about the strange, sweet smell that rivalled even the stench of decay? Some years later, I told the story to a mycologist — a fungi expert — at Massey University. He told me there was a species of fungus common in the soil called *Trichoderma* which smelled sweet, rather like coconuts. He thought that was likely to be the explanation, although he was at a loss to explain why it glowed in the dark. Perhaps, he suggested, it might be an undescribed species that could produce bioluminescence.

'Pity you didn't get me a sample,' he said. 'I would have loved to have examined it.'

Pity, indeed!

CHAPTER 3

The Naked Woman

Television programmes give the impression that pathologists spend all day opening bodies, weighing, examining then dissecting organs to find the cause of death. These cases are usually portrayed as part of a crime scene investigation, often with an unexpected twist. This may be true of dedicated forensic pathologists, but for the working pathologists in New Zealand's smaller provincial cities, life is quite different. Most days we work at our microscopes examining tissue biopsies of skin, breast, lung and bone, seeking evidence of disease.

It was mid-February, my first New Zealand summer. The rain drummed softly against the window. After growing up in Africa, it was a surprise to me just how wet and cold the weather could be in summer.

Twelve gastric biopsies since lunchtime and all were normal.

I felt myself succumbing to the monotony of it all — my eyes were trying to close and my head was feeling heavy —

when suddenly my friend and colleague James Pang came in and asked me to help him with an investigation. I looked up in anticipation. It was a welcome break. He explained that the police had a murder on their hands. My heart began to race. At last! Something new!

The case sounded nasty. A woman had been stripped and beaten to death in a paddock close to the control tower at the airport. Really? I looked out my rain-glazed window. I could see the control tower from the lab.

Within 15 minutes we were on our way. It wasn't difficult to find the place. There were half a dozen police cars parked on the verge of a small road on the outskirts of town, the usual sign of something seriously amiss. Emergency tape was strung about to keep the public out even though, thanks to the rain, there were few around to be the least bit curious.

New Zealand paddocks meant mud and cowpats. I should have bought gumboots, I thought, as cold water seeped through my shoes and socks. A policeman pointed the way across a fence. I made to climb over, but as soon as I laid hold of the wire, it felt as though someone had whacked my elbow with a baseball bat.

I yelled, leapt away, tripped and fell in an ungainly heap. I'd learned the hard way about electric fences.

I gathered the shreds of my dignity about me and squelched towards the far end of the paddock, where there was a cluster of uniformed and non-uniformed police.

Detective Sergeant Doug Brew introduced himself. He was a short, squat, hard-looking man with no discernible neck. His nose was fleshy and presided over by dense eyebrows. His complexion was plethoric and he redoled heavily of tobacco. His grip on my proffered hand was brutal.

'So the story is this. The husband says his wife didn't come back from the paddocks to pick him up from work. He phoned his son, who then drove down to the paddocks to look for her. He couldn't find her, so they phoned us.'

Doug was looking at us significantly.

'We didn't have too much trouble finding her,' he said, and gestured at the corpse.

The woman's body was stripped to her underpants and hung up in the barbed-wire fence. I recoiled mentally, although I was aware I showed no outward sign. Pathologists make mean poker players.

The body was covered with bruises, abrasions and dried blood. Her greying hair was heavily bloodstained. Her mouth was open and her purple, swollen tongue protruded from her lips. This was the picture of a brutal murder.

Doug walked us across the paddock, pointing out a trail of debris. There was a bunch of car keys, a stock stick, then a bra lying half-concealed in the grass. Much further on was a woman's top, the type of simple garment that could be bought at Farmers, the local department store. The trail led all the way from the body to the far side of the paddock. It didn't make sense. All I could suppose was that her attacker had ripped off her clothes as she tried to escape. We gazed across the farmland. A herd of Ayrshire cows grazed peacefully in the adjacent paddock. Overhead, there was a roar of engines as an elderly Dakota heaved itself from the nearby runway. I turned and looked at the control tower. It was clearly visible from where I was standing. To my mind, it seemed incredible that a person could be murdered in this wide-open space, in full view of traffic control. I didn't know an awful lot about the workings of the criminal mind, but it struck me that this was a most odd site for a sexual assault and murder.

I said so. Doug agreed. He looked worried.

* * *

Late that afternoon back at the mortuary, I helped Bruce lift the deceased woman off the gurney and onto the table. It was difficult as she was heavy and we are always gentle in our handling, not only out of respect, but also to avoid post-mortem injuries that could confuse the investigation.

There were many injuries, and of a pattern that seemed to indicate a frenzied beating. There were multiple fractures on both sides of the chest, and the sternum was fractured right through, a combination known as a flail chest. I had only ever seen this in high-speed motor vehicle accidents where no seat belt is worn and the steering wheel crushes the chest. This was the main cause of death. With multiple fractures to the ribs, the chest can no longer sustain the steady in-and-out motion of breathing. As a result, air entry becomes harder and harder and a death by suffocation invariably follows.

There was also heavy bruising to the breasts, as well as to the skin, muscle and fat of the upper part of the abdomen. The liver was ruptured and there was blood filling one-half of the chest. The blood loss explained her extreme, chalky pallor.

Doug Brew and his CIB team were watching carefully. He asked what sort of weapon would make these injuries. I told him that the only scenario I could imagine was one where she was trying to climb over the barbed-wire while her attacker was beating the daylights out of her with something very heavy. And not even a beating could account for the flail chest. It looked as though he had jumped on her chest with both feet or dropped his knees into her with his full weight; death must have been instantaneous.

'I've seen people beaten to death in tribal fights in Africa,' I said. 'I've seen men and women tortured and murdered by terrorists, but I've never seen anything as extreme as this.'

It didn't add up. I felt I was missing something. I wondered briefly what Doug was thinking. I had an uneasy feeling that he might know or suspect more than he was letting on. Whatever it was, he wasn't about to share.

My suspicion was confirmed when Doug returned just before eight the next morning. He told me he had decided not to open a homicide investigation and launch a manhunt for the perpetrator. His decision surprised me. I thought we must be dealing with a complete psychopath. And it was frightening that he was still out there somewhere.

Doug took James and me for a drive.

'I reckon New Zealand must be pretty tame after Africa?' Doug asked conversationally. 'I mean, you'd come across a lot of wild animal attacks over there, wouldn't you?'

'Actually, hardly ever,' I replied. 'Mostly the wildlife keeps out of the way of humans. Crocodiles take quite a few people, of course, but you never see them again. I did once see a man trampled by an elephant.'

I told him about the German tourist who had the double amputation in Kariba.

'Not likely to see anything quite like that here,' I said and laughed. 'Not many wild elephants around these parts. You're right. The bush seems pretty tame out here.'

'No elephants here, that's for sure,' Doug agreed. 'But sometimes you get surprises in this job.'

We pulled up beside a tidy, well-maintained stockpen. Tautly strung fences stretched out from the farmhouse, clicking softly as the high-voltage electricity flowed into them, keeping the stock disciplined and at bay. I was surprised to see the airport control tower not too far away. Obviously we had travelled in a large circle to get to where we were.

A grizzled, heavy-faced man, obviously the farmer, strode over to us. His complexion was scarlet with decades of sun and weather damage. Pearly keratoses and skin cancers were dotted along his broad nose and across his temple.

He extended an enormous, calloused hand — it too had a spatter of cancers over the back — and I braced for the inevitable crush. I was right to do so. It felt as if he habitually twisted number-8 wire with his bare fingers.

At some remark from Doug, he led us to the stockpen. I put my hands in my pockets and kept well back from the clicking wire.

On the other side of the fence was a bull, a stunning looking black-faced Ayrshire bull, a splendid, finely muscled animal with arching horns.

A bell began to ring in my mind. If Doug were showing us this bull, perhaps that meant that Doug thought the bull might somehow be involved ... Could the poor woman's injuries have been caused by a bull?

Bugger! Of course they could! That was the obvious answer. Why hadn't I thought of it?

I was feeling very foolish to have jumped straight onto the assault and murder bandwagon without having given as much as a thought to other possibilities. Injuries inflicted by animals can be horrific, and all the forensic textbooks have illustrative stories of injuries or damage to bodies caused by animals both before and after death. The lesson is that unwary pathologists should always think of animals when things do not add up. Of course, I was used to thinking of only wild animals, but stock can also be deadly.

A bull. Bloody hell!

James was nodding wisely, too.

'It's distinctly possible,' he said. 'The massive fractures of the chest wall could easily have been done by a bull.'

I cringed at how I had lectured the young policemen on precisely how the murder might have been carried out. I had even indulged a bit of speculation on the perpetrator's psychology — and all the while, Doug was watching me, quietly holding his peace. I could have crawled into a hole forever.

'So you think it was this bull?' I asked. 'What makes you think it was this one?'

'Well, I could see signs a bull had been in the paddock. I grew up on a farm, and I was always being told about how dangerous the buggers can be. There's a paddock full of cows over there. Reckon he probably jumped the fence to get at them. Plus the beast had been reported as taking an unhealthy interest in people.'

Doug lit a cigarette and squinted speculatively at the massive, sleek animal as it grazed peaceably. 'What about the clothes?' he said. 'How did the bull manage to undress her?'

Her husband solved the mystery for us. 'My wife was always pretty good with the stock. She told me that when a bull started getting aggro, the best way to deal with it is to take something off and chuck it on the ground in front of it. It distracts them. And while you're distracted, you can get away. Doesn't seem to have worked with this bastard.'

* * *

We had to have more proof to be able to draw a line and close the case. We decided we'd need to get some measurements of the bull's head, so that we could compare it to the deceased's injuries. We all looked thoughtfully at the animal. He must have weighed 500 kilograms. A vet was needed to dart him for us.

We returned to the mortuary and asked Bruce to bring the body out from the chiller. This time the approach was different. We carefully measured the exact size of the abrasions and bruises on the chest and abdomen, and looked at their pattern and how they might be joined. Quite quickly, it became evident that the pattern could well match a bull's head and horns.

The Cause of Death

The injury pattern in any assault often gives the size of the offending object. That, of course, is what we could and should have seen in the beginning. The eight and-a-half pages of meticulous description of her injuries told the story, but they also obscured it as effectively as any 'Where's Wally?' picture puzzle.

The bull was tranquillised, which gave us a window of ten minutes in which to measure the head and horns. The measurements were a pretty good match to the pattern and size of bruising. The bull was the perpetrator, without doubt.

* * *

Despite the ubiquity of farm animals in New Zealand, it's rare for stock to cause death. It was a decade before I saw another. One morning in the Horowhenua, a woman was butted in her chest by a rumbustious ram while she was bent over working with her sheep. A rib was snapped and the sharp, splintered end was driven into the back of her heart. It punctured the wall of the left ventricle — 12 millimetres of muscle — and then sprang back into position. Blood then slowly pumped out through the puncture filling up the pericardial sac and compressing the heart, thereby preventing it from beating. By the time she reached the ED in Palmerston North she was in extremis and barely able to breathe.

Richard Coutts was the surgeon on duty. He recognised there was only a matter of seconds left to act and no time to get to theatre. He opened her chest then and there, flicked the heart out and opened the sac, releasing the blood tamponade. He saw the puncture and inserted a deep stitch to close it off. Only then could the resuscitation and replacement of blood begin.

Initially all went well, but then her heart began to fail and it proved irreversible. I found at autopsy that the puncture and the stitch lay right next to a major branch of the coronary artery. The injury had sent the artery into spasm which stopped the supply of blood to the muscle of the heart. This effectively killed the heart muscle, causing myocardial infarction or a heart attack. Sadly, the heroic surgery, though essential, had not been enough to save her.

* * *

Even though we had identified the bull as the culprit in the case of the naked lady, two questions remained.

First, what should happen to the bull? It had proved itself to be a dangerous animal, but like the tiger in a zoo that kills its handler, it was neither more nor less dangerous than it had ever been just because it had killed. And meanwhile, it was valuable breeding stock. It was initially proposed that it should be de-horned, although that would have made only a marginal difference to the threat it posed. In the event, the beast was shot.

The other, and potentially more interesting question was how it was that the son had not seen the woman on the fence when he went looking for her.

Doug Brew had a theory. He thought it might have been a case of unconscious denial, where the mind simply cannot comprehend what it is seeing and so blocks it out. This might seem far-fetched, but I have actually seen a number of other cases of it. One striking example springs to mind. One of our lab technologists was killed in a head-on collision on her way to work. She was one of two women in the car. Both had fractured necks.

I arranged for our senior technologist to do the identification in order to spare her husband the need. The technologist took a long time looking over the dead woman's face.

'No,' he said. 'That's not her. But I know who it is.'

He named another technologist, who hadn't worked in the lab for years. But that woman was alive and well working in Hamilton.

When I checked the deceased myself, I found her to be clearly recognisable. The senior technologist's brain couldn't cope with the shock of seeing his colleague. He just could not bring himself to recognise her.

I was learning some strange but interesting lessons in the Manawatu. Real life was proving to be quite different from the textbooks.

CHAPTER 4

A Tale of Two Publicans

It may just be my shell-shocked view from the front line, but sleepy as the Manawatu and Whanganui districts are, we seem to have suffered more than our share of shocking, high-profile murders. I was centrally involved in two quite different cases, both strangely enough involving Manawatu publicans.

It startles New Zealanders to learn that there are about 50 or so murders a year — approximately one a week — in our green, bucolic splendour. It sounds terrible, but in the South Africa that I left, as many people were killed in a typical day as are murdered in a year in New Zealand. Back then, my country saw a murder committed every 28 minutes. So while New Zealand's homicide statistics are nothing to be proud of, it's very much a case of 'we don't know how lucky we are'.

Most murders in New Zealand are what the police refer to as 'name and address' killings, where the victim and the perpetrator already know each other. They include the well-known, hardy perennials — family killings, gang-related and criminal executions — as well as the tragically unexpected deaths, when alcohol- and drug-fuelled young men fight at parties and in the streets.

The common theme of these murders is the same, in that there is usually a body, which the police recover, over which the coroner takes jurisdiction and upon which the pathologist performs an autopsy. There follows a trial by jury and usually a guilty verdict, unless there is clear proof of insanity.

Meanwhile, though, the different categories of murder all occur out of different motivations. Family killings are often carried out thoughtlessly and in the heat of the moment, or occasionally as a result of severe mental illness. They include the murders of women — and sometimes their children — by their partners.

Criminal murders are usually cold-blooded and deliberate acts of commission, and gang murders are often part of an endless cycle of violence, not unlike warfare. The alcohol- and drug-fuelled fights are down to the addled loss of perception and the failure of empathy that follows.

The difficult cases are those where the murderer is unknown, the motive is unclear or the event is completely random. The difficulty is compounded when the murderer has no criminal record or known propensity for violence, and worst of all, is unknown to the police.

In such cases, pathology becomes vital. Evidence has to be methodically and painstakingly collected at the scene, in the mortuary and in the laboratory.

A Tale of Two Publicans

New Zealanders love to debate controversial criminal cases, and you'll often hear a case disparaged on the grounds that it was largely (or even wholly) based on 'circumstantial evidence'. This is interesting, because if evidence is weak, it is not the fact that it is circumstantial that makes it so. A very great deal of evidence presented in criminal trials is circumstantial, and it is often far stronger than eye-witness evidence, which is immeasurably more susceptible to human fallibility. Properly documented, circumstantial evidence can be unshakable. Pathologists often play a key role in murder trials, because in the end, pathology might almost be called the science of circumstance.

* * *

'Hi, Doc. Doug Brew.'

I had learned that whenever a call began like this, it would be interesting and probably harrowing.

'What can I do for you, Doug?'

'We've got a murder on our hands. We need you to check out the scene.'

'How do you know it's a murder?'

'Oh, pretty simple, really. The victim has had his throat cut. Sorry to bother you with it. I know it's your busy time of the day, but we shouldn't need you for long. Can you pick me up?'

I duly collected Doug in my ancient Daihatsu Charade, which I'd had shipped over from Cape to replace my crappy Toyota. As we drove through the farmland, basking in the summer sun, Doug filled me in on the scene.

The Cause of Death

The victim was Hugh Lynch, who owned and ran the Junction Motel in Sanson, 40-odd kilometres west of Palmerston North. He had been found dead in his office at the back of the motel by his wife early that morning. There didn't appear to have been a forced entry to the building, but police were nevertheless guessing Lynch had surprised a burglar, or vice versa. There had been a fight, during the course of which Lynch had been fatally wounded in the neck.

'Sounds pretty straightforward,' I said.

'Yeah, well. There's a couple of things that don't seem to fit. We'd be keen to get your opinion on them.'

Upon arrival in Sanson, my first job was brushing Doug down. I used my car every night to take Shumba, our golden labrador, down to the Manawatu River for a walk. She was a great shedder and Doug's jacket was covered in dog hair. It wouldn't do if Shumba's hair showed up in forensic evidence. These days, we put on surgical overgarments precisely for this reason. Back then, we did our best.

'Your warrant's out,' Doug pointed out as I beat clouds of hair from his jacket.

The Junction Motel was a flat-roofed weatherboard building standing at the intersection of the main roads heading north-south, and east-west. It was dark green, and had seen better days. Half a dozen police cars and the white unmarked incident investigation van were parked outside. Our arrival was noted by the constable on duty at the door.

The interior of the pub was dark and sad, but then most pubs look that way in the daylight hours. A detective was standing thoughtfully before a cigarette vending machine that was yawning open. A few packets of cigarettes lay scattered on the sticky, threadbare maroon carpet. A police photographer was kneeling to one side, pointing his lens at the machine.

I was given a more thorough briefing. Lynch lived on site with his wife and his teenage son. Lynch was quite a character. A local story was that he had won some money in the Irish sweepstakes years ago and had used his winnings to buy the motel.

The day before the murder, he'd had one hell of a row with his son.

Doug noticed my raised eyebrows.

'Nothing new about that. Most fathers and sons row with each other.'

I must have continued looked thoughtful.

'Of course, we're treating him as a suspect,' Doug added. 'We've taken him off to get a statement. If you've come up with anything you'd like to ask him, sing out.'

He pulled out his packet of cigarettes and lit one contemplatively.

'So Lynch seems to have locked up after closing time as usual, counted up the money and put it in the office safe. Looks like he was restocking the cigarette machine when the perpetrator somehow got in. There was no sign of breaking and entering, but the front door was probably open. It was definitely open when the milk delivery truck arrived just before six.'

I had already noticed a few odd things about the bar room.

There was a crumpled blue shirt on the floor. Doug saw me looking.

The Cause of Death

'That's Lynch's shirt. Apparently he always took off his shirt when he was about to have a punch-up or was chucking someone out of the pub. He'd peel off his shirt, come round from behind the bar, grab the offender and run them out the door. Looks like he decided to make a fight of it when he disturbed the offender.'

Lying on the bar-top was a blood-stained hand towel. That was the only blood in the bar itself. Doug then took me through to examine the body.

A narrow corridor led from behind the bar to an office. About halfway along the corridor on the wall and about 60 centimetres from the floor, there were intermittent, horizontal, faint smears of dried blood. It was an unusual pattern of distribution. It looked as though someone had lightly trailed bloodstained fingers along the wall.

The body was in the office lying halfway beneath the desk. The walls of the office were liberally splashed with blood — it was everywhere — and I instantly recognised the distinctive, sprayed pattern.

A lot of what happens in murder cases can be figured out from the blood patterns. Blood from the veins drips. Blood from the arteries sprays. And this was classical arterial spray, not only on the walls but all over the floor, the surface of the desk and even on the ceiling. All of the blood had been deposited in the same pattern. The deceased must have thrashed and struggled ferociously as he bled to death.

Lynch's head was beneath the desk and lying in a dark pool of congealed blood. There was a massive wound reaching two-thirds of the way around his neck. I could see the severed carotid artery, part of the thyroid gland and the larynx, which had been bisected. Glistening deep in the wound, I could even see the vertebral bodies of the spine. This was a spectacular murder, and far more than a simple slitting of the throat. This was a hemi-decapitation.

I examined the edges of the wound carefully. They had a distinctive, scalloped margin. I looked up at the under-surface of the desk. There was arterial blood sprayed all over here as well. I completed the examination as quickly as I could, noting in detail all these terrible injuries which I would have to describe in court later.

'What do you reckon?' Doug asked me.

'Do you have the murder weapon?' I asked.

'No sign of it,' he replied.

'I think you're looking for a bread-knife,' I told him. 'The pattern of injury indicates it wasn't a simple slash. His throat has been actively sawn with a serrated implement of some kind. Something like a bread-knife. Quite a lot of effort's gone into creating these injuries.'

'Defensive injuries?'

This was a predictable question. I had looked for these, too — injuries to the hands or arms that indicated the victim had tried to shield himself from the weapon. Defence injuries are always important in murders. They are invaluable in forensic pathology and are favoured by police, pathologists and lawyers alike. The police are keen on them because they are a strong indication that this is indeed a murder, and quite commonly where a victim has fought for their life, bits of skin or fragments of clothing torn frantically from the murderer may lie beneath the fingernails. Pathologists appreciate them because they give a further opportunity to identify the weapon from the pattern and type of injury, and it helps to establish the actions taken to avoid it. Lawyers also like them: the prosecutors because they reinforce the impression that death was the consequence of a deliberate assault; and the defence, because as soon as a messy struggle is involved, the chain of events becomes contestable.

'No defensive injuries,' I said. 'He's got blood on his hands. It's probably his, but his hands themselves are uninjured.'

'Where do you think it came from?'

'Well, it might have come from the neck wound, of course. But there's a bit of blood in his nostril. That might have got there from the neck, too, but I wouldn't mind betting he got a bloody nose from a punch in the bar. That would explain the bloodstained towel out there as well. And come to think of it, that would also explain the blood in the passageway. He might have got his hands bloody as he tried to stop his nose bleeding and his knuckles grazed the wall on his way in here.'

'Anything else?' Doug asked.

'There might have been two offenders,' I ventured. 'He was a big, muscular man. He obviously struggled like hell while they were sawing his throat open, but he had no defence wounds. I don't see how one person could hold him down and do the sawing at the same time.'

I finished my preliminary investigation and packed up. If all went well with the police scene examination, I would carry out a full autopsy the next morning.

A Tale of Two Publicans

Doug walked me out to the car, where a uniformed constable was examining my car and writing in his notebook.

* * *

The next day at 8 a.m., I performed a full autopsy on Hugh Lynch. There wasn't much to add to my findings from the previous day, which is often the case if you have done a thorough scene examination.

There it was then. A hemi-decapitation. A brutal, ugly, bloody murder. Pretty basic. Pretty feral.

It didn't take the CIB long to make an arrest.

Christopher Taunoa was a young man living nearby with his mother. When they arrived to interview him, the police found his mother's bread-knife with traces of Lynch's blood on the hilt. Some cigarettes were also recovered that were of the same brand and with the same distribution serial numbers as those that Lynch had been loading into the vending machine when he was murdered. And further enquiries revealed that Taunoa had banked a large quantity of coins in the kinds of plastic cylinders that were missing from the vending machine.

The police were pretty pleased with themselves. The court case ought to be a mere formality, given how meticulous they had been.

I could attest to their thoroughness. They didn't seem to have missed anything. I even got a letter through the mail that day alleging that I had driven my car without a current warrant for fitness, as deduced from the fact that it was parked at the Junction Motel on the day of the murder without displaying a current warrant.

* * *

A few months later, I was performing an autopsy on an 89-year-old man who had dropped dead while eating an ice-cream outside the local dairy. It was, according to police notes, a hokey-pokey ice-cream — vanilla ice-cream mixed with chunks of honeycomb toffee.

'Why did the police feel they needed to write this stuff down?' I wondered aloud to Bruce. 'Of what possible relevance could it be? Why are we even performing an autopsy?'

Bruce didn't reply.

It was a rhetorical question, because I knew the answer. It was bureaucratic. The man was very old. He had lived a healthy life, and his GP, who hadn't seen him for years, couldn't confidently sign a death certificate. The coroner had no idea of the actual cause of death, either, so a routine coronial post-mortem was requested.

We did a lot of these cases. We found that most of the deaths were due to coronary artery disease or a stroke.

'I sometimes wish I was French,' I told Bruce. 'They get to put "old age" as the cause of death.'

'That would cut down the workload,' Bruce said.

I agreed, but I pointed out that it also meant there was a certain degree of fuzziness in French mortality statistics.

'You know how the French are proud of maintaining they've a got a really low incidence of coronary artery disease?' I said.

Bruce nodded. 'It's all that good food and fine wine and' — he gave a Gallic snort of laughter — 'their passion for sex, isn't it?'

'Au contraire,' I replied. 'They just write off all their cardiovascular deaths as "old age".'

The phone rang. Normally the receptionists were careful not to disturb me while in the mortuary, so I knew it must be important. It turned out it was only a subpoena to appear for the case of *R* v *Taunoa*. I went up to collect it and understood from the officer that I would be in deep doo-doo if I did not attend.

The butterflies started flapping in my stomach.

The night before the trial, I took out my only suit — the same one I had bought for my final exams. It was absolutely necessary to wear a dark suit when appearing as an expert witness in court. I understood that this is not only out of respect for the court and the families of the victims, but it is also a mark of professionalism. I pulled out my scuffed shoes and a tin of polish and managed to coax them back to some sort of blackness.

I reviewed my notes and practised what I should say. Elayne had washed and ironed my best white shirt and sponged a tie, which she pressed to a crisp newness. She was both excited and impressed that I was to be a witness in a murder trial. I didn't tell her just how nervous I was feeling.

Just before I was due to leave for court the next morning, I picked up my daughter to give her a hug. Vicky beamed happily at me. I swung her up above my head and brought her down for a cuddle. She then vomited a gush of semi-solid, sour milk down the front of my suit.

Elayne fetched a damp cloth. She rubbed until the fluff stood up on my jacket, and the milk stain, thankfully, seemed to disappear. I sped along the road, anxious not to blot my copybook by being late for my first court appearance. I needn't have worried.

I waited outside the courtroom for half an hour. A detective from the CIB came out. He looked over at me, his eyes lingering on the milk stain, which had staged a ghostly reappearance, nodded and walked out of the court house. I waited another half hour. The foyer was filled with heavily tattooed men in none-too-clean denim and dishevelled women wearing track pants. The women easily matched the men for the number, coverage and exuberance of their tattoos. Footwear varied from jandals to scuffed biker boots. The air was coarse with the reek of tobacco.

These people were grist to the mill of the justice system, all awaiting their call before the bench. I eyed them, idly wondering what they were here for. They eyed me back, especially the men. My suit and briefcase were noted. There was a mild hostility in the air.

Eventually I was rescued by a young woman lawyer who took me through to the public prosecutors' room.

Here I waited. And waited.

This is a feature of the court system that I would come to know very well: the long hours of sitting, waiting in court. It's always slower than you'd think possible.

I waited.

Eventually the door to the little room burst open and Ben Vanderkolk, the Crown Prosecutor for Palmerston North, strode in. He is tall and broad, a lawyer with a larger-than-life personality. He was wearing a voluminous black gown and a wig that seemed a couple of sizes too small for him.

'Right. So you're the pathologist on *Taunoa*,' he said breezily. 'Have you done this before?'

I confessed I hadn't.

'Nothing to be worried about. All anyone wants you to do is give your evidence.'

We quickly went through my deposition, Ben asking pertinent questions from time to time to clarify points of detail. What sort of knife was used? Why did I think that the knife was serrated? How much force did the murderer need to use to saw through the victim's neck? Those were the critical pieces of evidence he was going to have me present to the jury.

Ben's junior brought in a tray of cups and a pot of coffee. She smiled encouragingly at me. She had removed her wig. And while I was wondering where the wigs were kept, I noticed my shoe. The toe was splashed with Vicki's regurgitated milk. I glowed with embarrassment, but I didn't have a handkerchief or anything else I could use to remove it. And now that I had noticed it, I was acutely conscious of it, as though it was a bright beacon announcing to all and sundry that my grooming — and, by extension, my professional standards — were highly suspect.

I gulped down my coffee and was shown through to the public gallery of the High Court and seated in a chair at the front.

The Cause of Death

It was my first time in a courtroom, and I looked around with interest. The high seat where the judge was to sit resembled a panelled wooden pulpit and was directly in front of me. Above it, hanging on the wall, was the New Zealand Coat of Arms. I noticed for the first time that this features a yellow-robed Maori warrior holding a staff facing a young, blonde Caucasian woman, barefoot and dressed in angelic garb. Both are standing beside a shield emblazoned with sheaves of wheat, a flotilla of mediaeval-era ships and what looked suspiciously like a sheep carcass suspended from a hook.

I made a mental note to try to find out what it all meant later.

There were two prison wardens to the side of the main body of the court and in front of them stood a solitary, sullen-looking man. He wasn't all that large although he was quite muscular. He was dark-complexioned and plainly anxious, shifting from foot to foot. I stared, fascinated. This was the prisoner. Could he really be the murderer? That neck, sawn virtually in two by *this* man?

I shook my head to clear it. It wasn't for me to decide. I had only to tell my part of the story. Then it was up to the jury.

The bewigged officers of the court began filing in.

Standing to the left of the judge's chair was a man in a black and white robe. He suddenly called out: 'Come to order, please, ladies and gentlemen. The Court is in session. All rise for Her Majesty's Judge.'

We all stood up.

A Tale of Two Publicans

An elderly, robed man wearing the most magnificent wig of all entered through the back door, stood before his seat and bowed three times, once to the left — it wasn't clear to whom this was directed — once to the centre, in the direction of the Crown prosecutor and counsel for the defence and the accused: they all bowed back, with the notable exception of the accused and the warders, of course, who all stood staring fixedly ahead. The last bow to the right was definitely to the jury. The foreman of the jury, a thin, middle-aged man bowed back. Was I expected to bow, too? God only knew what the protocol was supposed to be.

I sat quietly and watched. And while waiting, I studied the sea of legal wigs assembled. They were all quite different from each other. They varied in colour from pure white to a pale lemon, perhaps faded by age. Some were blandly simple and functional; some were fuller, with combed tracks through them, and one or two had a curious little pony-tail appended. They were all perched rather precariously on legal heads. I wondered how they stay there.

There was discussion between the prosecutor and the judge, and then between the defending counsel and the judge. I couldn't hear any of it, because they mumbled at each other. Eventually, I was called and installed in the witness box and the judge asked the court crier to administer the oath.

Ben Vanderkolk led off, smiling encouragingly at me. His questions were easy. He took me through the murder scene, painting it in stark pictures for the sake of the jury and the judge. He then led me through my findings. And all the while, I was quite convinced that Ben was staring intently at the milk stripe on my suit as he spoke, willing it to disappear.

I was asked about the severity of the attack and how I would rate or grade such an injury. I described the hemi-decapitation and the considerable force required to carry it out. A few small noises from their direction indicated that this news was uncomfortably received by the jury.

And then Ben handed me over to the defence lawyer, Duncan Harvey. His questions were well thought-out and cleverly constructed, as one would expect of a man who was to become a respected judge. The first questions were easy, matters of fact only. No opinions were needed or asked for. But gradually, the questions changed and became more and more probing. I realised he was taking issue with my description of the type of knife involved. I had expected this, as the typing of knives from wounds is far from a precise science. Defence lawyers have a field day with subjective matters such as that.

Harvey built up his case meticulously, question by question. I was quite sure he was building up to asking the inevitable question: whether one young man alone could have perpetrated such an atrocity. But for whatever reason, he never did, even though Taunoa cruelly tried to implicate Hugh Lynch's son. That was shown to be quite impossible.

Finally the judge turned towards me and said: 'Very well, Doctor. Thank you for your assistance here today. You may go.'

And so I left my first homicide case.

A Tale of Two Publicans

Somehow I didn't feel I had acquitted myself quite as well as I had hoped. But as Elayne pointed out, I was limited in what I could achieve by the questions put to me.

In the end, Christopher Taunoa was found guilty and sentenced to life imprisonment. He had 19 previous convictions, including some for violent crime. The jury were unanimously convinced that he was the sole perpetrator, although I still wonder to this day where he found the strength to carry out this terrible murder alone.

* * *

I remembered Hugh Lynch and the Junction Motel one Monday morning a couple of years later when I arrived at the mortuary. I was greeted by Ian, one of the mortuary assistants.

'Good morning, Doctor,' he said. 'Dr Darby has one autopsy this morning and he would like your opinion, please.'

Dr Roy Darby was a doyen of pathology in the Manawatu. He had been the lab director in the Palmerston North Hospital laboratory for years and in fact, was instrumental in recruiting me to my position. Roy was officially retired but he had hung onto his practising certificate and helped ease our workload enormously by performing large numbers of the routine coronial cases. He had made it clear he didn't want to deal with suspicious deaths or homicides, as he'd had a gutsful of court and cross-examination in his time.

The deceased was a publican from a small hotel on the Wellington Road. Dr Darby gave me the facts.

The Cause of Death

'He's been found at eight o'clock in the morning lying on the floor of his pub with his head in a pool of blood. He was unconscious, but alive. He's been taken to ICU [the intensive care unit] and they've treated for an embolism [a stroke]. He's been on a ventilator for the last eight days, but he died last night. I'd be grateful if you'd have a look. It doesn't smell right to me. What's the external bleeding all about? I'm not satisfied it's natural causes.'

I read through the huge pile of notes, observations and hourly blood tests meticulously documenting the man's last eight days of life. Everything was charted, controlled and monitored. I could see his steady decline as he'd drifted inexorably to death. It was all there, minute by minute, hour by hour, and day by day. It seemed straightforward on the face of it.

Nonetheless, like Dr Darby, I felt uneasy. I was deliberately trying not to draw a connection with the other publican, who had been so savagely done to death in a different pub, 40 kilometres away. I had seen many strokes, but never one with external bleeding.

The story from the constable, first at the scene, was sparse and unhelpful: 'An unconscious man was found in a pool of blood, breathing irregularly. An ambulance was called, an urgent trip to the hospital arranged.' That was it. When the anaesthetist in charge of the ICU called the police to announce the publican had died, the death was referred to the coroner, who had ordered a post-mortem. Not much to go on there.

The problem became evident as Roy and I carried out the autopsy. The scalp was opened from ear tip to ear tip with a scalpel and peeled forward down over the eyes to expose the gleaming skull.

'There we go,' said Roy.

The right side of the skull was shattered with a depressed fracture of the parietal bone. The whole bony cranium was shattered and pushed into the underlying brain. The injury wasn't even small. It was the size of a beer bottle. There had been bleeding into the tissues of the scalp, causing massive bruising. And I could see these injuries had been there a good while, at least eight days.

We opened the skull by sawing a circular cap from the top of the head, a process almost exactly like taking the top off a boiled egg with a spoon. We lifted the hard dome of the skull, exposing the soft brain beneath.

I wasn't surprised at what I saw. There was a massive extradural haemorrhage. The fractured skull had torn the middle meningeal artery where it lay in a groove in the skull and this had bled out. The resulting blood clot was trapped beneath the hard bony skull and as it grew, it exerted more and more pressure on the brain. The bleeding would have been progressive over several days until the thrombus — the blood clot — began ramming the brain down out of the skull into the bony spinal column. This would have been fatal, instantly fatal, as the nervous centres responsible for breathing are compressed and fail.

But I knew at a glance that this was not a stroke in the sense of a bleed due to medical causes. This was a traumatic death, due to an accident, perhaps, but also quite likely due to an assault, even a deliberate murderous act.

The Cause of Death

Roy and I peeled off our gloves, chased a surprised assistant out of the mortuary and locked the door. I picked up the phone and dialled the number for the CIB.

I told the person who answered who I was.

'We've just performed a post-mortem on a man who died in hospital last night after suffering a traumatic brain injury eight days ago. Based on what we've found, I think it's a matter for you guys.

'Eight days ago?' the policeman said. 'Ah, shit.'

* * *

Within half an hour, Doug Brew and his homicide team were in the mortuary glaring down at the partially dissected remains of the publican, as if they could force the truth from the corpse with sheer belligerence. Doug was annoyed at the possibility that a monumental mistake had been made and a murderer might have an eight-day head-start.

'How the fuck did the hospital miss this? Stroke, my arse,' Doug grumbled.

The detectives all looked at me.

It was a reasonable question. I had asked the radiologist to come down to the mortuary to review the imaging with me. We had looked at the CAT scan images, and he had pointed out the fracture on the scan that was done on the day the publican was admitted. The duty radiologist had simply missed it. In the absence of any imaging evidence of a fracture, the doctors had made a clinical diagnosis based on the victim's symptoms. It was wrong, and there were tragic consequences. Had the fracture been identified at the time, an emergency trephine could have been performed to lift the fractured skull off of the brain. He could have been saved.

'If this is murder, we've got our work cut out for us,' Doug said. 'Can you tell us anything about how he came by this injury?'

'Well, he's suffered a heavy blow to the side of the head. It would have to be something weighty …'

'A fist?'

'No, I don't think a fist could do this much damage. A full beer bottle, maybe. Maybe a fist, if the guy was big enough.'

'What if he was hit multiple times?'

'Not likely,' I replied. 'He would have tried to defend himself, but there are no defensive injuries. No, it's more likely he was hit once and hard and that put him down.'

The CIB headed off to examine the scene and collect statements about who was where and who knew what. Our job seemed easy by comparison. All we had to do was determine a cause of death, and we'd done it. They not only had to find a murderer, but also sufficient evidence to convince a jury of guilt.

A week went by. Then Doug phoned and asked if I would meet him in the pub. Roy Darby decided to tag along. He might have been over presenting evidence in court, but he clearly hadn't lost his professional curiosity. His pathology instincts were like an old warhorse sniffing blood and pawing the ground.

'So what we've learned is that the publican was found first thing in the morning by the day staff. He was lying on the

The Cause of Death

floor next to a bar stool in a pool of blood. He was still breathing, but irregularly. The staff called an ambulance and, of course, the police. The local constable who lived on the far side of Palmerston North attended.'

'I know all of this from the notes,' I said.

'Yes, but get this. The bar stool was next to a table, and on the table were three plates. On each plate there was a hamburger, chips and tomato sauce bought from a local take-away. All three burgers were half-eaten, about the same amount each. There was also $1500 in cash, all stacked in piles by denomination, fives, tens, twenties and fifties. These were stacked up on the bar in full view. Nothing else.'

Roy and I looked at each other in amazement.

Three people sharing a meal, one has a stroke and topples off onto the floor, so the others just put down their burgers and go home? How likely was that?

The investigating constable didn't think it was odd. The money was still there, so there couldn't have been a burglary. No burglary, no crime, see?

Unfortunately, the whole place had been tidied up on the morning of the incident. The hamburgers were thrown out, the plates were washed and industrial cleaners were brought in to get the blood from the carpet. By mid-afternoon, the whole place was as spic and span as it was likely to get and was ready to serve customers again that night. The money had been banked and was now untraceable.

Doug said the police had questioned anyone who could be even so much as remotely involved. It was clear that the deceased had picked up an order of three hamburgers and chips from the local take-away, but he did so alone. He chatted for a few minutes with the owner of the place, but there was no-one else waiting with him and he didn't give any indication who the other two hamburgers were for. No-one saw him leave the pub and go to the take-away, and no-one saw him return. The trail, in short, was stone cold.

'What I'd like to know from you,' Doug said, 'is whether you think a man falling from this stool,' he patted it, 'could sustain a fracture like the one our guy had on his head.'

I examined the scene carefully. The bar stool was of standard height and the floor was carpeted.

'Well,' I said, after I'd thought about it. 'I'd say it's about as likely as the idea that one man would eat half of each of three meals. After all, men in bars fall from their stools quite often, but I've never come across this particular type of injury before. What do you reckon, Roy?'

'Quite right,' Roy nodded.

Doug ran his fingers through his hair in frustration. We all knew it was unlikely there'd be a breakthrough in this case. There may have been a crime, there may not have. The money might have been a couple of nights' takings. Doug thought it was unlikely to have been a drug deal, as those didn't happen in the Manawatu back in 2003. That sort of money is more likely to have been used for gambling on horses, but if anyone was flashing those sorts of sums around at the races, the police would likely have heard about it. The money was a dead end, too.

The investigation was closed, and the death pronounced to be the result of an accidental fall. I had always held the naive belief that the police left no stone unturned until they got to the bottom of things. So much for that. We had to agree in the end that there was no evidence to suggest anything else.

Whenever I walk into a small-town pub, and am greeted by the man behind the bar — rough diamonds, in a lot of cases, but invariably friendly and welcoming — I think about these two cases. There's an abiding, nagging dissatisfaction, the sense of something unresolved about both of them. It's as though their ghosts are leaning on the bar beside me, still waiting for their answers.

CHAPTER 5

A Touch of Madness

The more calls I received from the CIB, the more I came to enjoy the unexpected, the unusual and the challenge that they heralded. I took to keeping a 'murder bag' in the boot of the car, holding all the stuff — gloves and instruments and sample jars and so on — that I might need, as well as waterproof gear and tramping boots. I knew now not to touch rural fences without a swift glance along the strand of wire for plastic insulators.

This call came one day at mid-morning. The scene was out of town in an isolated house near Pongaroa, a good two hours' drive away on dirt roads from Palmerston North in the southeast of the lower North Island. We met at the police station in Dannevirke before proceeding to the scene. There were half a dozen police cars parked outside. Doug Brew was there with his team, along with the locals. It was a tight squeeze, all those bodies in that little police station.

The Cause of Death

I met Jerry Cray, an enthusiastic local officer who had made the discovery. Jerry Cray was late twenties, curly blond hair and prematurely balding. He was large, athletic and competent. You had to be competent to police these extensive districts.

'I got called to go to a rural address. The resident is a male person in his fifties, a bit of a recluse, really, and he regularly has stuff delivered — groceries, cigarettes, that kind of thing. But when the delivery guy went to drop the box off this week, the previous week's box was still there, untouched. He called me. I drove out there and inspected the box and the house.'

He paused, as if for effect. Brew, who was leaning against the wall listening, waved his hand in a coaxing motion.

'Jerry, Jerry. Why are you doing this to us? Tell us what you found!'

Jerry hastily obliged. It was thought the deceased had lived most, if not his entire life in the house in which he was found dead. He had no income besides his benefit, which was banked and out of which his weekly supplies were paid for by automatic payment. He had no relatives, at least none were known. He never left, and everything had basically decayed around him.

'It's bloody unbelievable. You'll see what I mean when we get there. It's shit-full of garbage. Anyway, his body is lying on the bed and he's been shot between the eyes. There's a bullet wound right here,' he pointed to a spot between his eyes. 'Reckon it's a .38 calibre.'

'Anyone else live over there? Any ideas who might have done this?' Doug lit a cigarette, concentrating on the flame.

'Nah, there's no-one around here would do anything like that. I mean there's the young chap, Sam. He is a bit of a tearaway. But a good kid at heart. He'd never do this sort of thing. I have to knock him back every now and then, but he's okay. And there's a bit of weed smoked but not much else goes on.'

I got the distinct impression that Jerry was the law around here and kept everyone more or less in line. That's the way it worked in small, rural communities.

Doug puffed on his cigarette and grinned through the smoke. 'Come on, Jerry. Take us up there and let's take a look at this gunshot wound.'

* * *

It took us another hour on roads that grew ever narrower to reach the house. We drove past paddocks full of sheep mustered for shearing. Men and horses and dogs were out working the flocks. The Ruahines shimmered in the distance. It was a beautiful afternoon.

As we approached the house along its narrow, unkempt driveway, long grass swishing under the floor of the car, the signs of pastoral prosperity evaporated. The house itself came into view, and you could see that it had been quite grand in its day, standing amongst spacious, well-tended gardens. You had to imagine the gardens, now. There was a flat area alongside it that might have been a tennis court, or even a croquet lawn. It was anyone's guess. Regenerating bush had reasserted itself, and gorse and scrubby manuka were growing right up to the door.

We walked to the door. The air was close and humid. Jerry stopped.

There was a dead black-and-white kitten lying in front of the main door, which was standing open. I could see the cat was partly mummified, and I guessed it had been dead for quite some time.

'That bloody cat was not here this morning!' Jerry said. 'I swear that's true for absolutely bloody certain! That cat was not here this morning!'

'Jerry, don't do this to me,' said Doug. 'Next thing you'll be saying it's witchcraft.'

We stepped over the carcass and soon forgot about it. The hall leading from the front door was stacked floor-to-ceiling with garbage. There were thousands, perhaps even tens of thousands, of empty tins, every one of them identical: baked beans tins. There were collapsed cardboard boxes, sodden newspapers and thousands of bottles, all lemonade bottles, all a single brand. There must have been decades' worth. The stench was more a taste than a smell. And the whole mass quivered, rattled and clinked as hordes of rats burrowed, scratched and feasted within. Every now and again, we caught glimpses of rapid movement, of pink, scaly tails snatched out of view as we turned to look.

As I walked gingerly along the narrow alleyway between the towering stacks of rubbish, I glanced into the open doorways. The rooms were all the same — all stuffed with subtly moving rubbish.

It was easy to find the body. That one clear passageway led from the front door to where the body lay on a bed that had been set up in what would once have been a formal lounge room. That, too, was filled with garbage, a mountain of it threatening to cascade in an avalanche over the bed. The man might have been asleep were it not for the smell, which even over the putrid smell of the rubbish announced to me that decomposition had set in. He lay on his back, his legs crossed. He was fully clothed in dark but dirty attire. A rancid-looking toe stuck through a hole in his custard-coloured, crusty socks. His unlaced boots lay untidily beside the bed. His arms were also crossed and in his right hand was a cigarette that had burnt down to the filter and then extinguished itself. The ash remained, a 30-millimetre-long column lying on his chest.

His sightless eyes stared up at the ceiling. Small white eggs — blowfly eggs — flowered at the corners of his eyes. On the bridge of his nose, right between the eyes, as Jerry had said, there was what appeared to be the entry wound of a bullet, likely .38 calibre.

I turned to look at Doug. He was shaking his head in disbelief.

I examined the body carefully. The deceased was obviously resting peacefully while holding a lighted cigarette in his fingers when he died. Clearly, then, he hadn't been disturbed. Any murderer trying to make his way from the front door through the trash canyon would have found stealth impossible. The noise we had made was enough to wake all but the deepest sleeper. So how had he been shot so neatly between the eyes, apparently without any warning?

I delved into my murder bag and came out with my magnifying glass. I felt faintly ridiculous. I could almost feel Doug's lip curling, as though he was expecting me to also produce a deerstalker hat.

I examined the injury around the bullet wound. It was blackened about the edges, the classic sign of a bullet discharged at point-blank range: the blast from the explosion tattoos the edges of the wound distinctively with gunpowder residue. I scraped the edges of the wound with a scalpel blade to collect carbon particles and tapped what I had gathered onto a glass slide. Forensic scientists could examine it and confirm the presence of soot and cordite.

Nothing came off the blade. I examined the wound again through my magnifying glass.

There were strange, vertical streaks radiating from the edges. The streaks were parallel and evenly spaced. The bone in the centre of the wound gleamed, clearly intact. I tapped lightly on it with the tip of my ball-point pen to be sure. It was solid. No bullet had ever entered through here.

If this wasn't a gunshot, what was it?

Then I spotted his earlobe. It was puce with rot. And yet it looked surprisingly tatty. I examined it under the magnifying glass. There were strange similarities to the wound between the eyes. Here were the same parallel scours, the same thin abrasions raking through the decaying skin. Now I knew what it was.

A Touch of Madness

I stood up and turned towards the detectives.

'Well?' Doug said.

'This isn't a gunshot wound,' I said emphatically.

'So what's the verdict, Doc?' he asked.

'Rats,' I replied. 'All of the injuries here have been caused by rats. I'm not sure what the actual cause of death is, but I'm quite certain it'll prove to be natural, once I have done an autopsy. He's clearly died here peacefully, lying in his bed. This injury which you see has been caused since by rats feeding on his body.'

We all looked at the rubbish. It still clinked and shifted furtively around us. The rats didn't care about our presence: they knew they were safe, dug in deep in their festering rubbish. We all shuddered.

Rats always go for the soft parts, such as the earlobes, the lips and the eyelids. This case was unusual only because some persistent rat had gnawed away at the unpromising, bony spot between the eyes. Other than that, the parallel marks of the rat's teeth on the wound between the eyes and on the earlobes were absolutely typical of rat predation on the dead.

We lifted the body onto a stretcher with some difficulty because of the closely packed rubbish. While trying to be helpful, I stepped back, lost my footing and fell with a crash into the high cliff of cans and bottles. They cascaded all over me. Everyone laughed sympathetically.

I carried out an autopsy the next day. There was no problem here. There was a thrombus, or blood clot, in his left anterior descending artery. He had suffered an acute myocardial infarct, or heart attack. That was completely consistent with the cigarette ash indicating a sudden, peaceful death. A close look at the injury between his eyes confirmed it was superficial. There were very well-defined tooth marks at the edges of the wound, obviously those of a rat.

I phoned Jerry Cray to tell him and was surprised to hear that he was going to torch the place. He thought it was a health hazard and a disgrace to the district.

In an odd sequel I told my colleague Bruce Lockett the story and said I thought it was a pity it was going to be burnt down as there might be some valuable old furniture in there, given the age of the house. Within minutes Bruce had Jerry on the phone and convinced him that the two of them should go through the place first. Half an hour later, Bruce was off to Pongaroa. An afternoon of hot and sweaty work shifting years and years of rubbish revealed only a pedestrian kitchen table, made from an unidentifiable and entirely unmemorable timber. There was nothing of any value whatsoever

For months afterwards — and in the years since — I have often thought about this sad, lonely life and wondered what drove the man to live life as a recluse. Was it really his happy childhood home? Could he ever have imagined his lonely death and that the house would end up a fireball? It was yet another window that death occasionally provides into the strangeness of human lives.

* * *

I thought I had pretty much seen everything when I saw the trash palace, but a matter of a few weeks later, I was involved in an even more bizarre case. I had sat up till late watching television. Elayne and the children were long asleep and I had staggered off to bed at 11.30. I had been asleep only an hour when the phone rang. I sat up, gasping, trapped for a moment in that awful place between dream and reality. Anyone who regularly takes medical calls at night knows that place.

'Hello? Hello?' I croaked into the phone. 'What do you want?'

It took me a while to make sense of the call. I didn't recognise the voice, and all I could gather was something about a body and a locked room. I had to ask the caller — a policeman, as it turned out — to repeat himself several times before I began to understand. A body had been discovered in a locked room. The circumstances were inexplicable. They needed a pathologist's opinion on the cause of death before they knew how to treat the scene.

I asked the policeman on the end of the phone for directions, which was a mistake. I simply lacked the encyclopaedic knowledge of the history, geography and the current retail activity of the city that his complicated description presumed.

To further complicate matters, it was pouring with rain. It was only after methodically searching the poorly illuminated backstreets, peering through the streaming windshield, that I eventually found the house.

It was semi-detached, one of a group of houses companionably clustered on one side of the street and built by a developer in the 1970s. I could see several darkly clad men standing underneath the carport out of the rain. I parked and made a dash to join them.

I recognised a detective from the CIB.

'Morning,' he said.

It did not feel at all like morning to me. It was more like a very bad late night.

'I'm sure this is a murder,' he explained. 'I'm afraid we can't go in at the moment, because the photographers are taking pictures. We'll have to wait a few minutes.'

We stood waiting in the carport while the rain pelted furiously onto the roof and overran the guttering. It was cold and a wet mist swirled around us. Ten minutes. Twenty minutes. Half an hour passed. I began to shiver.

While we waited, I studied the car with which we were sharing a shelter. It was an immaculately kept, old veteran car — a heavy, 1950s sedan, a Vauxhall Victor, complete with sun visor above the windscreen. I hadn't seen a sun visor since the early 60s. The paintwork was unblemished, the hubcaps gleaming. I peered through a sparkling side window.

Lying on the dashboard was a pair of driving gloves, left on right, thumb to thumb, finger to finger, perfectly aligned. A period map box sat in the centre of the front bench seat. The car clearly belonged to an unusually particular, perhaps even obsessive-compulsive individual. I wondered whether he was a mortuary assistant.

After what seemed an age, the detective in charge joined us.

'Sorry to keep you waiting. A fuck-up with the photographer. Let me tell you about it.'

The rain slashed angrily around us.

'The deceased was in a back bedroom, which was locked with the keys on the inside of the door. He was identified, and was the registered owner of the property, no criminal record, nothing known, not even a fucking speeding ticket. Well, that wasn't a surprise. Look at the car. Every door to the house was locked, also from the inside, and all the keys were present. There was no evidence of breaking and entering.'

He went on to say the house was peculiarly tidy and it was clear nobody else had been in there. Yet it looked as though there had been a serious fight in the room in which the body was lying. The puzzle was: how did the perpetrator get in or out?

There was one other piece of information, which may have been significant, or it may have been a distraction. A conman, well-known to police, had been working the area that night with one of his old scams. What he did was ring or knock furiously at a door, late at night, when people were in bed and already asleep. When they answered, he overwhelmed them with bullshit. He said something along the lines of: 'I'm John, your neighbour. You know, next door. My daughter in Whanganui has had a serious accident and is in hospital. I've got to get over there right away. But I need money for petrol. Can you lend me $20?'

Apparently it usually worked. In the 1980s, most people were still fairly trusting. Many didn't know who their neighbours were, but they would nevertheless hand over the money and forget about it until the next morning.

But that night was different. A neighbour was suspicious and had phoned the police. The conman was picked up and the murder was discovered when the police decided to check out the other houses along the road.

The conman was locked up at the station, where he was apparently looking very sorry for himself. He had been told he might be charged with murder. The detectives, by contrast, looked grimly satisfied.

I went into the house. The front door led directly into the lounge room. I stopped in astonishment. I'd never seen anything like this before. It seemed that any present the deceased had ever been given was carefully arranged on the surfaces of the house. Every mantelpiece, every table, every surface was heavy with toys in pristine condition. There were Dinky cars, model aeroplanes, train sets, board games and jigsaw puzzles, some still partially wrapped in the original birthday and Christmas paper, some unwrapped but still in their boxes. Some of the presents still had tags: 'Happy Birthday to a good boy' and 'From your Uncle Thomas and Aunt Mavis. Happy Christmas 1961'. The writing on the labels was formally spaced and elegantly written in royal blue ink with a fountain pen.

Here we go again, I thought. This is going to be about psychiatry. I was good at recognising the signs and causes of death, but I couldn't begin to fathom the kinds of behaviour in a life like this. If I couldn't understand what was going on in his life, then how was I supposed to find the truth about his death? I knew I needed to understand his story.

The door to the only bedroom had been opened. A police locksmith stood to one side, nodding at us.

This room was different. It was an absolute shambles. The bed, bedside table and lamp had been turned over. Shards of glass from the shattered lightbulb glittered on the carpet. The bloodstained bedding lay all over the room. The mattress was on the floor and a pale, glistening foot stuck out from beneath it, the shin protruding from the cuff of blue striped pyjamas.

Every book had been pulled from the bookcase, spines split, pages ripped and hurled around the room. There was more blood on the books. Even more appalling were bloody handprints and even footprints up to a metre above the floor and covering every wall. There was even a handprint, beside other specks of blood, on the ceiling. The central ceiling lamp was intact, but the shade was hanging awry. Everything seemed to speak of a huge and ultimately fatal battle.

But how did it happen? Who had done this?

The window was intact, the door locked. The only certainty was that it had ended with a corpse. I inspected the foot, which was bloodstained. There was a small cut in the ball of the big toe, not nearly big enough to be fatal, and definitely not a 'defence wound' from an overwhelming attack.

I flogged my brain, trying to recall anything I might have happened upon in a textbook that could explain a scene like this. I could think of nothing. The only thing I felt able to eliminate was the involvement of any wild or domestic animal. I had learned that lesson well enough.

'Are you quite sure the door was locked?'

The police were adamant. The scene had been discovered by a very reliable constable. He saw the body through the window, which was locked. The police locksmith confirmed he had a bugger of a job to get the door open from the outside. There was no other way in or out.

The Cause of Death

I knew this couldn't be a murder. Everything was against it. The locked room absolutely excluded it. I considered a bizarre form of suicide. Roy Darby had often spoken of a research biochemist who had injected himself with snake venom, but how improbable was something like that? I couldn't come up with any likely scenario.

Usually autopsies are done as soon as possible so that homicide investigations can get underway. We all looked at our watches: 2 a.m. We all were in agreement this couldn't be a murder, so the scene was locked up and a constable placed on guard. The body would be uplifted and brought to the mortuary for an autopsy first thing in the morning.

We all headed off to bed. I puzzled all the way home. There must be a precedent somewhere, an answer in the huge wealth of forensic cases and literature. But I was buggered if I could think of it. I certainly wasn't going to think of it at two o'clock in the morning.

I sank into bed. The windows rattled abruptly in their frames, the floor shuddered and then subsided. The ceiling light swayed. A minor earthquake juddered past. I looked up uneasily. I was getting used to these, too. Probably only a magnitude three or four. Bugger all really.

Life in the Shaky Isles goes on.

* * *

The autopsy was tricky — not technically, because that part was easy. It was tricky because, despite a meticulous dissection, there was absolutely nothing to find. This happens surprisingly often in post-mortems. About one in ten of all of our cases fall into this depressing category. The pathologist can find nothing. We reported those out as 'obscure natural causes' — or, to put it politely, we have no idea at all.

The autopsy was made more difficult in this case by the presence of CIB detectives. Their professional scepticism hung in the frigid air with the odours of death. They were sceptical that there was nothing to find. Sure, there was a deep cut on the vascular ball of the right toe, but I'd seen that last night. And as it turned out, that one cut was the source of the entire, bizarre pattern of blood splattered about the room.

But there was no pulmonary embolism, the vessels to the heart were normal, there was no aneurysm, and there was no stroke. He hadn't been strangled to death. He was entirely normal in every way, from a post-mortem perspective. In theory, he should still be alive.

But if any case cried out for an explanation, this was certainly it.

'So what are we calling it, Doc?' one of the detectives asked. 'Natural or not?'

'I just don't know the answer to that,' I said. 'The best I can offer is that toxicology might have something.'

Deep down, however, I was just about resigned to a verdict of 'obscure natural causes', which wouldn't bring anyone any satisfaction.

* * *

The Cause of Death

I had collected blood from the femoral vein in the leg as well as from the liver, kidney and brain. I also took samples of stomach contents and bile from the gall bladder, and everything — neatly packaged and labelled — was sent off for toxicological examination.

It was a few days before the results arrived.

Two drugs were found in the blood from both the femoral and cardiac specimens. One was haloperidol, an antipsychotic drug. The second was promethazine, also an antipsychotic drug. The trouble was, both were found only in sub-therapeutic levels.

I thought hard.

Two drugs, both to treat the same condition? Why two, when only one was needed? And why were both at a low — effectively useless — level? I couldn't see a logical answer to these questions, so I picked up the phone and called the psychiatry ward in the hospital. The deceased must have got his antipsychotic drugs from somewhere.

The deceased was unknown to them, so he must have got the prescription medications from his general practitioner. I discussed the case with the psychiatrist, but she too had never heard of anything like this before.

The lab results had arrived on the Friday. The answer came unexpectedly on Saturday morning.

I had mowed the lawn, played with Richard, read the newspaper — all the things I liked to do on my day off. I had idly picked up my copy of *MIMS* (the medical reference book published annually but once known as the *Monthly Index of Medical Specialties*), and turned to 'Pharmacology: Indications,

Interactions and Side Effects'. I paged desultorily through it. Then, out of curiosity and because it had been much on my mind, I turned to the index and looked for haloperidol, the first drug found in my subject's blood. There it was. And there were pages and pages of side effects.

Blood dyscrasias — what the hell was that? — liver disorders, skin rashes ... More of everything and anything that any drug could, and from time to time did, cause. I yawned. But as I was closing the book, the words at the bottom of the page caught my eye: 'Neuroleptic Malignant Syndrome'.

A thrill of adrenaline ran through me. I had it! It was rare, so very rare, but I had found the solution!

'Neuroleptic Malignant Syndrome,' I read, 'is a rare disorder manifesting usually when a patient under treatment for a psychotic disorder is changed from one neuroleptic drug to an alternative neuroleptic drug. In the change-over phase when both drugs are at relatively low levels, some individuals may idiosyncratically manifest the Neuroleptic Malignant Syndrome.'

So what was this bloody syndrome? I turned the page and rapidly scanned the words.

'The patient develops serious visual hallucinations, becomes extremely fearful and will attack all objects both animate and inanimate vigorously. The patient is almost impossible to restrain and will particularly attack mirrors, windows or glass, wherever there is a reflection. Extreme pyrexia (fever) may ensue, followed by arrhythmias of the heart and sudden, unexpected death.'

The Cause of Death

This had to be it! It explained the strange findings and now I was sure this case was no longer murder. Who had changed the deceased's medication? Probably his harassed general practitioner, some poor bastard just doing his best, no doubt, and who, like me, had never heard of Neuroleptic Malignant Syndrome. Deaths from medications do occur, but they are extremely rare, especially in the provinces.

Further investigation confirmed it. The deceased man's GP had apparently recently changed him to haloperidol and stopped his previous medication. Somewhere before the old meds had faded from his bloodstream and before the new meds had kicked in, he suffered a bizarre, unpredictable and very rare — one in a hundred thousand — reaction. Someone has to win Lotto. Someone has to be hit by lightning. And someone has to have a rare drug reaction. That day, the spinning wheel of chance decreed that it was the turn of the man in the locked room to die.

The CIB were over the moon. They hate unsolved mysteries even more than I do.

* * *

Death from prescription medicines is rare and this was the only such case I have come across. They tend to happen in hospital when patients are in dire straits and need aggressive treatment, such as for cancers. I have also seen two cases of death from alternative medicines and herbal remedies. Just because they are 'natural' doesn't mean they are innocuous. Many are not safe, and their oversight is non-existent compared with pharmaceutical medicines — as I found out while investigating a tragic case.

It involved a woman in her late sixties who was being treated for diabetes. She'd heard a radio advertisement for a herbal tonic and decided to give it a go. She developed severe diarrhoea but persisted with a lower dose on the advice of the agent who had sold it. The diarrhoea persisted and she became so dehydrated that her kidneys failed. She had been careful to continue both her conventional and alternative medicines. Unfortunately, her meds included Metformin for her diabetes, which came in a blister pack, one for each day of the week. Metformin is excreted from the body in the urine and of course, this can no longer happen if the kidneys are failing. The net effect was that she accumulated lethal quantities of the drug in her blood, which became so profoundly acidic that even the expert management she received in ICU could do nothing for her.

The herbal tonic contained 13 different herbal ingredients including cascara, bladderwrack and the naturally occurring compound anthraquinone, which is found in rhubarb leaves. All of these can cause diarrhoea, and although it is impossible to find absolute proof after death, the timing suggests to me that she died a victim of a lethal cocktail of natural and conventional medicines.

Of course, natural medicines do not have to interact with conventional drugs to kill people. They are perfectly capable of doing it on their own. I was asked to carry out a 'hospital' autopsy on a patient who had died in the ICU. Hospital autopsies used to be very common and many, if not most, people who died in hospital were autopsied. It was the bulk of our workload back in the 1980s. The hospital doctors, young and old, revelled in these and the chance they gave them to quite literally learn from their mistakes. But such autopsies virtually never happen now. Perhaps we don't make mistakes anymore.

This was an unusual patient; he was an overseas academic on a sabbatical visit to Massey University. He unexpectedly went into kidney failure and despite the best efforts of the specialist staff, he continued to decline. He was repeatedly questioned for any information that might explain this catastrophic turn of events, but he couldn't help. He soon passed away.

I found nothing. The autopsy was boringly normal, the toxicology was uninspiring. I sat at my microscope to look at his tissues with a heavy heart. Heart: nothing. Brain: nothing. Lungs: nothing. Pancreas: nothing. Kidneys: nothing.

Wait!

Just as I was about to toss the kidney slide away, I sensed rather than saw a peculiar texture to the tissue. It wasn't obviously abnormal: it just wasn't quite right. I looked more closely. There was something in the tubules. It was so nearly completely transparent that I almost missed it. I polarised the light and the kidney lit up like a firework display, a cascade of luminescent and subtly coloured crystals crammed into and blocking every single tubule. No wonder he couldn't make urine. No wonder he was in renal failure. No wonder he died.

But what caused these crystals?

Analysis soon revealed they were oxalate, or oxalic acid. Some babies are born with congenital oxalosis but he was far too old for that. I knew you could get oxalate poisoning from drinking antifreeze. Ethylene glycol, the active ingredient in antifreeze, is a complex alcohol that can produce intoxicating effects similar to ethanol, or ordinary booze. Thousands of drunks give it a go each year in the United States, but it's fairly toxic stuff. It turns into oxalate crystals and gums the kidneys up tight. You'd have to be a destitute alcoholic to give it a go and even then, it would be (quite literally) your last resort.

So not your usual Massey academic, I thought.

There are other, rarer causes. Peanuts can do it, in very large amounts. That seemed improbable, too. He would have to have been throwing back massive handfuls of them, day and night.

The eventual answer came as a surprise. Apparently he had read how antioxidants in the diet were the fashionable favourite to prevent atheroma and coronary artery disease as well as most types of cancer. These fads are usually fanned by the press, who promiscuously shift their approval around, from blueberries one day to Brazil nuts the next and everything in between in the meantime. Mostly the claims are rubbish. Vitamin C was the compound du jour, and the deceased thought: well, if a little is good, more must surely be better! He ate industrial quantities of vitamin C — thousands of grams every day, compared with the one to two grams you need to maintain healthy levels — and he died

The Cause of Death

as a result. Vitamin C is toxic in large amounts. It causes oxalate crystals to precipitate out, and they set in the kidneys like concrete.

The job occasionally throws up ironies such as this. The shortcut to death was the vain pursuit of a longer life.

CHAPTER 6

Drug Mule

It seems that everything in my life starts with the phone ringing. Death knocks and opportunity, of course, does the same, but for pathologists it is always the ringing phone that signals disaster has befallen someone. In this case, the call came late one Sunday afternoon when I was in the middle of my siesta. As usual, I felt drugged with lassitude from my afternoon sleep, and I had to concentrate hard to accurately jot down the details of the scene to which I was being directed.

By the time I had driven the 45 kilometres to the intersection of State Highway 1 with Pioneer Highway and Highway 56, I was more alert. I found the scene easily. It was marked, as usual, by the multi-coloured swarm of police cars, like wasps around windfall fruit.

In the midst of it all sat an elderly, two-toned, orange and grey Anglia, parked at a careless angle by the side of the road, as if it had run off the seal and coasted to a stop in its own time. The driver's door was open and out of this protruded the elasticised cuff of a pair of grey stretch track pants and a bare foot. This was why I had been summoned.

I didn't know the detective in charge. He told me they were following up an inquiry from the Asian Crime Squad.

I looked quizzically at the body. He was about 35 years old, blond and definitely Caucasian. 'Yeah, I know, the detective said, as though he'd read my mind. 'The "Asian" bit is a hangover for the days when all the drugs came from Asia. The Asian Crime Squad is the National Drug Squad.'

Drugs! This was very unusual. In the 1980s and 1990s, Palmerston North was hardly a centre of the international drugs trade.

I examined the body more closely. A plume of frothy blood had oozed from both nostrils and from his mouth, and had formed a clotted pool encrusting his hair and forehead. I could see no injury from my first, superficial inspection. A spilled carton of milk lay on the floor. His arm was folded over his head, his fingers stretched out as if in supplication towards the spilled milk.

On the face of it, the death looked peaceful.

I learned that the Drug Squad had become involved when they received reliable information that a considerable shipment of cocaine was being trafficked from Australia into New Zealand, which was regarded as a soft touch in those days. They thought it was going to be flown into Wellington and then held in the rural backblocks.

I wasn't sure whether I should be offended at the description of the Manawatu as a rural backwater.

Drug Mule

'This guy fitted the typical profile of a drug mule exactly,' the detective explained.

'In what way?' I asked.

'He's young, he doesn't have much money — he's a research assistant in his day job — but he takes a short trip, a couple of days, to Australia. When he comes back, he looks jittery and he's trying to get through Customs in a big hurry. We searched him and his possessions, but we didn't find anything.'

He had evidently been travelling from the airport later that same night when something had gone wrong. Here he was lying dead, half in, half out of his car on State Highway 1 for everybody to see. Dozens of cars passed him and not one reported the odd-looking scene to the police. Instead, someone contacted a local talkback radio station, and six hours before the police found his body, the entire listening world heard there was a bloke sleeping half out of his car on State Highway 1 close to the Himatangi turnoff. The DJ made a couple of jokes at his expense, but no-one thought to investigate.

It wasn't until a police patrol car happened by that the death was discovered.

I had read about drug mules who attempt to smuggle cocaine across borders by swallowing condoms stuffed with the drug. The condoms occasionally burst in the bowel, releasing instantly lethal doses into the bloodstream. I had never seen such a case myself and was quite excited at the prospect of performing a post-mortem on one.

* * *

The Cause of Death

A full gallery of policemen were in attendance, seated behind the protective Perspex screen in the viewing area above the dissection table. The screen was to stop spectators being splashed with bodily fluids. An autopsy is a very liquid experience.

I gathered a few of the younger ones hadn't seen an autopsy performed before, so I was determined to make it a good one for them. They watched attentively as Bruce, whistling through his teeth, used long-bladed garden secateurs to split the deceased's rib cage on either side of the sternum. The bones crunched as the blade sheared through each rib. His whistling stopped as, with a grunt, he snapped the sternoclavicular joints, then he lifted the breastbone backwards. It parted from the lungs and heart beneath with a sound not unlike tearing tissue paper.

'There you go, Doc. All ready for you.' He stood back.

I took a scalpel and drew it firmly down the front of the abdomen. The rectus muscles of the abdominal wall peeled aside as the yellow and purple intestines, distended with gas, bulged into view. Quickly I dissected the larynx free, releasing the great arteries of the head, neck and arms and peeled the thoracic organs out of the chest. The body lifted off the table as I pulled, but only briefly. As the organs lost their hold on the spinal column and tore free, it slumped back again. I cut around the diaphragm, pulling upwards and outwards and peeled the abdominal organs out in one continuous pluck. All that remained was for me to detach the bladder and rectum through the lower pole of the prostate gland. All the organs, other than the brain of course, were now free. I lifted the entire mass onto the dissecting table, which took some effort. It weighed around 50 kilograms.

The watching detectives looked impressed. One or two looked a bit green.

I turned the organs over and picked up a pair of scissors. In one, practised sweep, I peeled the oesophagus open past the larynx, right down to the oesophago-gastric junction.

'Any time from now,' I said, looking up at the detectives. 'Any time from now we should come across the condoms.'

I opened the stomach. There was only curdled, clotted milk inside. It smelt — well, it smelt like curdled milk, sour and unpleasant. I scooped it out with my fingers into a pot. It would be sent for toxicology analysis. There was nothing else there.

I continued to cut through the pylorus and into the duodenum. The condoms must be in here, I thought.

There was nothing there, either.

I opened the entire gut from end to end. I worked hard and fast, pulling loop after loop of shiny intestines through my hands as I opened them, squeezing out the semi-digested food within. The smell of bile, sour digestion and wet faeces rose into the air.

One of the detectives, a thick-set, dark-hued, middle-aged man with a thin upper lip, gagged, turned and stumbled out, pushing through his solid mates. His complexion had gone a curious, greyish blue. Bruce regarded the poor chap's vanishing back with lips pursed in disapproval. He followed him out. He didn't want any mess on his mortuary floor.

The Cause of Death

The remaining policemen laughed and joked — a cover-up, no doubt, for what they were all feeling.

I completed my investigation of the alimentary tract. I shook my head. This was no drug mule. But what had killed this otherwise healthy looking 35-year-old man? I had recently handled several cases in which the cause of death was reported to the Coroner as 'not ascertained' or 'obscure natural causes'. I hoped this wasn't going to be another one.

It should not have been a surprise that a late-night hunt for cocaine in a provincial mortuary was going to be unrewarding. I looked up speculatively at the gallery of police. I could see they were as disconcerted as I was at the false trail. Cocaine was their mission: the cause of death was mine.

I peeled the spleen off the pancreas and it slithered out of my gloves onto the weighing tray of the mortuary scale. I noted it was normal at 122 grams. I cut it in half, and it was diffluent, liquefying into a consistency not unlike sewerage as it began to decay, but there was no cause of death here.

And finally I held his heart aloft like some Aztec priest. It was a large, dripping, pigeon-sized double handful — a big pigeon, at 285 grams in weight. Spread over the surface of the heart, matching the course of the underlying coronary arteries, were constellations of perfectly formed, star-shaped haemorrhages, one beside the other, trekking from the origin of the artery in the aorta, over the surface of the heart and into the muscular substance of the heart itself.

'These are what we call petechial haemorrhages,' I told the policemen. 'Beautiful examples, really.'

'What do they mean?' one asked.

'Well, they're not a specific pointer to any particular cause of death. I've seen a lot of different conditions causing them — sudden heart attacks, fatal irregular heartbeats, cot deaths. You occasionally get them in cases of murder by strangulation.'

That got their attention, but I pricked that bubble straight away.

'He definitely wasn't strangled. These marks along the lines of his coronary arteries indicate a sudden death, but apart from telling us it was sudden, they don't tell us anything else.'

I took all the usual specimens of blood, urine and liver for toxicology analysis. But in the end, it looked likely to remain a mystery.

But as I was nearing the end of my investigations, I heard the bell announcing that someone was entering the mortuary. There was some rearrangement amongst the detectives in the front row, and suddenly there was a constable standing there. He had some information.

'I've just come from visiting his gran,' he said, nodding at the dissected remains of the man. 'She's been expecting him for the last day or so.'

The detectives were staring at him. I could tell it wasn't disbelief. They believed him only too well. Their expressions were of the 'Oh no. Have we fucked this up?' variety.

'He told his gran he was going to be back late Saturday night, maybe Sunday morning, because he was going to drive through from the airport directly. He never arrived.

She'd made him a roast leg of lamb on Sunday, thinking he was delayed and would come later. The story checks out. I saw the lamb myself.'

And then he dropped a bombshell.

'Oh, and he's a diabetic.'

Diabetes!

Suddenly it was clear to me. I hadn't thought of that possibility. At his age, he would have to have been an insulin-dependent diabetic, so surely there must have been syringes, needles and insulin in his luggage. Once the police checked again, there were. It turned out these items had been overlooked in the excitement of chasing up the cocaine trail. Besides all that paraphernalia, there was a diary of doses and times of injections. The answer was there if only they had looked for it.

When I later studied the diary, I found that the last entry told the whole, sad tale. He had landed and was in a hurry to get through Customs because he knew he was overdue to inject himself with his early morning dose of insulin. Once he'd done that, he'd headed out into the darkness and set off driving towards his grandmother's house, three hours away. But he hadn't eaten. He had little glucose in his blood at that hour and an injected bolus of insulin pushed it even lower. Then one by one his brain cells began to die.

Somewhere along the road he must have realised what was happening, pulled the car over, and scrabbled about anxiously trying to find something to eat. The best he could do was a quarter-pint carton of milk. There is lactulose in milk, but not glucose. It was something, but not enough to stave off disaster. He probably knew this as he made his last, futile effort to live. He must have gulped the milk and then collapsed across the seat. The brain cells kept dying and so, in due course, did he. He was dead of accidentally inflicted, fatal low blood sugar — an incidental victim of international travel, if you like.

Diabetics know that a meal must, simply must, follow an injection. Fatal hypoglycaemia will certainly follow if no food is taken. He ought to have known better, but I have found accidental death is often the result of miscalculations and 'what-ifs'. His was a pointless, avoidable death, as they go, but that is usually the problem with revisiting the past. It's so easy to be wise with hindsight.

I was disappointed I hadn't been able to hold up a ruptured condom fished from the ileum of a drug mule. The police came out of it fairly crestfallen, too, but no-one had suffered anything by comparison with the man's broken-hearted family.

CHAPTER 7

The Devil Comes to Town

'Good evening, this is the six o'clock news brought to you by Judy Bailey and Richard Long. Today in Palmerston North police announced that one of their constables had been tied up and mutilated in his own home. The home was then torched, apparently by devil-worshippers, in the most serious home invasion seen in New Zealand to date.'

Thankfully, the constable was still alive. But hysteria was growing, fanned by excited reports, each one less believable than the last. Devil-worshippers? In Palmerston North? That seemed ridiculous. The news had been breaking throughout the day. Civic leaders who should have known better also fanned the flames saying there was growing evidence of active devil-worship in Palmerston North. There was talk of Satanic rituals, and Nelson MP Nick Smith called for a ban on violent films, seemingly convinced there was a link between the attack and a similar scene in the movie *Reservoir Dogs*.

Children were in tears at school and the Ashhurst community, where the attacked constable, Brent Garner, lived, was in the grip of fear. Police were wondering who was next. Those out on patrol in the surrounding districts were issued with pistols to be worn at all times — a first for New Zealand, let alone the district.

Palmerston North was getting into a fine old froth.

* * *

Doug Brew asked me to look at Brent Garner's injuries.

Doug gave me the background story. I sensed he was irritable. This attack had surely pissed off the police and they were out for blood.

'The short story is this. Brent Garner lives in Ashhurst,' he said, 'a small settlement of about five thousand people 14 kilometres out of Palmerston North. He's received in the post three hate letters threatening death. Nothing unusual about that. Most police are pretty well used to this sort of thing. You know, the odd burglar you've picked up, a domestic you're investigating, even the odd rapist — they all send you hate mail from time to time. These ones were by post, letters cut out from a very large variety of magazines and stuck on a page to make a message — just like the movies. It's still pretty effective and hard to track. Especially as the magazines used had no theme.'

I saw copies of the messages. The job of cutting around the letters had been neatly done, giving the impression of being unhurried but not obsessional. They were all cut in much the same way with about the same margin around each. Each letter was stuck more or less neatly in a line, meaning it was probably done by one person. Everything looked pretty tidy. The message itself was simple, but literate. It was obviously the work of a person who was still functioning well, not of some tense psychopath.

I was particularly interested in just how naive the hate letters were. I would have expected at least some degree of sophistication from devil-worshippers: after all, they must have thought about it, studied it and found something to attract them to the cult. I could see no evidence of intelligence, and there were no passionate religious or even anti-religious sentiments here.

Brent was a tall, young, dark-complexioned man with compelling blue eyes. He had not shaved since his ordeal, and had advanced stubble, dark, rough and irregular. He looked at me, tired and anxious, when we arrived. I smiled reassuringly. I examined Brent's back. I had never seen the like. I had seen some pretty flamboyant and cruel mutilations during the war in Africa, but this was, well, different.

There were long, deep cuts, both vertical and horizontal, across his lower and mid-back. They were surprisingly straight. Some people had decided they were a crude pentagram, which was said to be an emblem of the occult and, if inverted, represented Satan and evil. I couldn't see any such pattern. My conclusion was that people were so obsessed with the idea of the devil that they saw what they wanted to see.

When we got outside, Doug asked me if I thought the wounds could be self-inflicted. I didn't think so. The cuts were definite and unwavering, applied without hesitation. There were no 'practise cuts' anywhere. I have often seen practise cuts on wrists or throats in suicides, where the victim is afraid it will hurt and has a few goes before making the final, fatal deep cut. But you never see practise cuts in a murder. Murder is committed in a rage, usually fast and furious. One, maybe two deep cuts and the job is done. Not lots of little attempts before the big one.

Although this was not a murder, I thought a vindictive devil-worshipper would not have held back. His or her cuts would be more like these, straight and made in a sweeping slash. I couldn't imagine any way that every single cut could be so long and relatively straight if you did it yourself with your hand twisted behind your back.

I was pleased to hear that Richard Coutts, a general surgeon, had also examined Brent's injuries and had reached the same conclusion.

I asked Doug what he was going to do and he was characteristically blunt.

'I am going to catch the fucker that did this and I'm going to lock him up!'

* * *

I heard later there were some worrying aspects to the case. There had been an alarm system in place at Brent's house and it was linked directly to the nearby Ashhurst Police Station, but it had been mysteriously disconnected at the time of the attack. By whom? Who had both access and motivation? No-one knew, but it had to have been someone at the station.

And then there was the matter of the dog. I was reminded of Sherlock Holmes in *The Silver Blaze*:

'*Is there any point to which you would wish to draw to my attention?*'

'*To the curious incident of the dog in the night-time.*'

'*The dog did nothing in the night-time.*'

'*That was the curious incident,*' *remarked Sherlock Holmes.*

Brent's usually vociferous dog Max was silent throughout the invasion and attack. Why was that?

Doug was sufficiently suspicious to set up a secret parallel investigation to Operation Venus, the team who were investigating the offence. This was code-named Operation Mars and was headed by Grant Nicholls.

I was asked to accompany the Mars team to the Garner home in Oak Avenue in Ashhurst to see whether we could re-enact Brent's dramatic escape. We all met outside the partly gutted house early one morning. There were a number of detectives present whom I did not know as they had been drafted in from other centres to keep the team secret. Besides me, there was also a short, lithe, tightly muscled man with no discernible neck.

The introductions over, we moved inside the shell. There was a rank smell of charcoal and wet cloth.

We were told that Garner was in the lounge room when the assailant burst in, overpowered him, bound him hand and foot and then gagged him.

The wiry little man in our midst was introduced. I was

surprised to hear he was an escape artist of some sort. He must have been recruited from a circus.

I was asked to tie him up with plastic garden tie-locks to recreate Garner's account of events. The escapist stripped off his shirt and denims. He was incredibly muscled, not bulky like a body-builder, but each muscle was perfectly defined. He could easily have been used for an anatomy demonstration, like one of those carefully flayed corpses that were once used to teach medical students. He lay on his stomach on the charred carpet and with the help of one of the detectives, I pinioned his arms with his hands pulled up between his shoulder blades. I wrenched his hands as high as I could, just as the photographs of Brent Garner had showed. I thought it would be painful but if so, the escape artist gave no sign. His legs were trussed equally as tightly.

The detective and I stood back and studied our handiwork.

'He's not going anywhere fast,' the detective said.

During the attack, both the room and Brent were liberally doused with petrol. The intruder then walked down the passage to the front door, a distance of eight, say nine paces and that was all the time Brent was out of his sight. It was only a few seconds, and that's all Brent had to get clear before the house was torched. Brent said he had managed to drag himself across the floor to the open window and throw himself out just as the fireball erupted. He was lucky that the window was wide open — although that, too, was odd, because all the windows were supposed to be secure because of the threats.

The window was quite high off the floor, and while the escape sounds straightforward it certainly was not so. As soon as he was given the signal, the expert rolled rapidly across the room and with several extraordinary contortions got himself on his knees hard up against the wall. I would have said it was physically impossible if I had not seen it myself. It had taken eight seconds.

But here, he was thwarted. Up and on his knees was as far as he could get. He tried even more extraordinary manoeuvres: his contortions became even more fantastic. He even tried to throw himself off the floor at the window. He hurled himself at the window and crashed face-first into the wall. It was a heavy impact and I was surprised his nose didn't start bleeding. I wondered if I should help him, but the stopwatch was still running.

He surrendered. It was impossible.

I cut his ties. The poor chap looked crestfallen.

'Can't be done,' he said tersely. That was his professional opinion.

To be sure, we repeated the whole exercise, this time using a constable of the same height and weight as the tall Brent Garner. I trussed him up in much the same way. He didn't do nearly as well, managing only to roll to the window. Even that was accomplished with great difficulty, and he was quite unable to get himself up even marginally off the floor. At least he didn't crash face-first into the wall.

* * *

It was perplexing. We met up in the old public library in Palmerston North to decide what to do next. As well as

Grant Nicholls and the Operation Mars detectives, the police psychologist, Ian Miller, was present. He was a specialist like me, but of the mind and not of the dead.

There was a distinct sense that we needed to complete this investigation quickly and successfully. The rhetoric in the press was that the whole business was an unpleasant reflection on the country; to my mind, and I think most of the police shared my opinion, it was ridiculous.

Ian Miller gave a succinct and intelligent appraisal of the probable mental status of the perpetrator. He had some interesting information to share about Satanic worship, which apparently was practised by a small number of fairly average people, all quite normal in every other way but for this unusual mental ideation.

We glanced at each other in surprise. None of us had any idea there really was such a thing as devil-worship, and to think it was being secretly practised by our apparently normal neighbours ... well, that just goes to show you never know what goes on behind your neighbours' doors. Maybe the city councillor wasn't so out of line as we had all so derisively supposed?

I was then asked again whether the cuts could be self-inflicted, but I stuck to my guns. I still thought they must have been put there by someone else, and for the same reasons. But now, since we had demonstrated that it was impossible to escape from the house as Brent had described, the chances were that he had an accomplice, as he had either had help escaping or he was tied up only after leaving the house.

The Cause of Death

Things moved quickly, and after protracted interviews, Brent made a full confession. He had staged the whole thing. He was absolutely insistent that he had acted alone so that he could give the insurance payout on the house to his wife. It turned out he was having an affair with a typist who worked at the police station in Palmerston North, and he planned to separate from his wife and marry her.

He was adamant that his injuries were self-inflicted and that he had escaped from the burning house. And he never changed from this position. So maybe I was wrong all along. But I have always wondered what happened to the balsa-handled scalpel that Brent said he used to inflict the cuts. Perhaps the handle was consumed by fire but the blade should still have been there. As far as I know it was never found.

Interestingly, a nearby resident reported hearing someone running down the street shortly before the fire broke out at 4 a.m., but he couldn't provide any further details as he didn't get out of bed to look.

It was a good outcome. At least the armed policemen were off the streets and all the talk of evil undercover Satanic cults dried up. But it was a colossal waste of police resources, having cost $350,000.

Brent Garner pleaded guilty and was sentenced to five years in jail. He was an exemplary prisoner and was released after serving a third of his sentence. He drifted a bit but sadly was unable to come to terms with life. He was found dead in his car one morning near Matata. I don't think he was a bad person, although on any analysis, his choices were pretty flawed. He paid a very high price.

The Devil Comes to Town

* * *

Sometimes, things happen where a supernatural explanation seems simpler than the reality. Take the case of the man cooked in his car. Here, I saw something that very few pathologists have ever seen, and indeed, something that many do not believe exists.

Doug Brew had asked me to come out to a puzzling death out in the countryside. I drove out with a couple of my registrars; these are the young doctors who train with us to become pathologists. Their training runs for five years.

We drove past broad paddocks filled with quietly grazing Romney sheep until we eventually came across a blue Mazda pulled over at an angle on one verge, with a police patrol car pulled over on the other, Doug Brew standing monumentally beside it.

As we got out, I looked across at the blue car. The windows were strangely opaque and grey, and there was what I took to be a blurred face pushed up hard against the rear side window, which was partly open.

'Member of the public called this one in,' Doug told me. 'The car belongs to a local man from out Foxton way. He comes across most nights to drink in Sanson. He was there last night. Left at midnight, pretty pissed, from all accounts. Only thing of note in the car besides the body was a bottle of spirits which he probably got from the bar.'

'Isn't that illegal?' I asked.

'Yeah, but it happens,' Doug frowned.

'And this isn't the road to Foxton,' I pointed out.

The Cause of Death

'Yeah, well, he seems to have got out of his way. Probably disoriented on account of being pissed, ended up here and decided to cut his losses and sleep it off in the car.'

'What happened then?'

Doug tossed his cigarette butt in the roadside ditch.

'That's what I was kind of hoping you'd tell me,' he said.

I crossed the road and cautiously opened the driver's door. I reeled backwards, gagging, as I was assaulted by the smell. Pathology acquaints you with some pretty choice aromas, but I had never smelled a stench like this before. It wasn't the smell of death and decay. This was somewhere between truly rancid fat and some sort of low-grade paraffin with a sulphurous tincture of eggs, all mixed in the worst possible way. I gasped for breath, trying not to retch. (Curiously, I lost my sense of smell some years after this, after contracting dengue fever in Fiji. It has been an asset in my line of work at times, and it would have been a boon that day.)

Eventually, it either cleared a little or I became more used to it. I steeled myself to look inside. I was flabbergasted. On the back seat was a body, the upper two-thirds of which had been badly burnt. Much of the body was just blackened, congealed fat. Both arms were similarly reduced yet the left hand was clean and undamaged without so much as a scorchmark.

Apart from that hand, the recognisable remains of the body were the right side of the face, which had been resting against the rear passenger window, his lower pelvis and legs. There were absolutely no signs of burning to these areas and even more bizarrely, there were no scorch marks on the upholstery of the seat nor on the head-lining above. The windows were clouded with greasy soot but that was all, despite the massive burns to the body.

I thought I knew what this was, but I didn't quite believe it.

'This,' I announced to Doug and to my registrars, 'looks like a case of spontaneous combustion.'

The others looked at me blankly.

I explained that it is a very rare condition — if, indeed, it exists at all. In these cases, the body apparently just bursts into flame and yet there is little or no burning anywhere around it. It has been reported for centuries. Back in 1725, a French innkeeper's wife, Nicole Millet, was found burnt to death with only cinders remaining. The innkeeper was charged with murder and sentenced to death. He was pardoned after he convinced the authorities that this was a spontaneous immolation and clearly a visitation by God. Others who claim to have witnessed cases would reject that defence, as they are convinced it is the work of the devil.

Such scientific opinion as there is to support it suggests that it usually happens to alcoholics. Their bodies are typically found — as ours was — melted away with no damage to anything around them and no obvious source of ignition. The most likely explanation is that the alcoholic is either dead from other causes or has been rendered unconscious by drink, whereupon something as insignificant as a burning cigarette starts the process. It lights the clothing which chars the underlying skin and melts the subcutaneous fat. The fat, saturated with alcohol, is absorbed into the clothing, which sinks into the body and acts as a candlewick. Tallow candles, which are made from animal fat, work in exactly this way. And so the cycle starts. As the fat burns, the fluids are burnt off and eventually even the muscle and organs may be consumed.

I thought perhaps our victim had pulled over as Doug suggested and amused himself drinking his bottle of spirits before crawling over into the back seat to turn in. At some point before losing consciousness, he had lit a cigarette, and this has fallen, still alight, onto his clothing.

I thought the half-open passenger window would admit enough air to feed the flame without fanning a huge fire. It would be a typical 'wick effect'. When I read up on it later, I found this exact sequence has been reproduced in experiments using a pig carcass.

It's curious that the car seats and interior didn't burn. This is because the burning body is exactly like a candle. You can try it. Put your finger right next to a candle flame and you'll feel nothing. Nothing beside it or around it will burn, but it's plenty hot enough inside the flame to keep melting the wax and to keep the wick glowing. The body fat, too, keeps burning until eventually the whole body is melted and turned into soot. When the fat is all used up the flame gutters out.

The same research I read indicated that the dreadful smell is characteristic, as is the sparing of the hands and feet. The 'candle' burns until it reaches the hands and feet. There is no fat stored in the extremities, so in a classical case the feet and hands often fall off totally undamaged and are found unscathed beside what is left of the rest of the body.

'So,' said Doug flatly. 'An accident, then.'

Typical bloody cop. No sense of scientific occasion whatsoever.

'And there's one thing I don't get,' he added. 'Why is the car pointed towards Sanson and not Foxton?'

I shook my head. I didn't have an answer to that. Typical pathologist. No matter what you discover the police always have one last unanswerable question.

CHAPTER 8

In the Arms of Ecstasy

Pathology is a little like Forrest Gump's box of chocolates, 'You never know what you're going to get.' I found the apparently infinite variety that the job threw up a source of constant amazement. By the time I had been working there for a couple of years, I realised that I actually loved getting to the mortuary in the morning.

Bruce Scott was always at work long before I arrived to make sure that everything was perfect. One morning he came into my office and dropped a bundle of forms on my desk.

'Got another dead in the arms of ecstasy, Doc. You get them from time to time.'

'What do you mean?'

'You know. In the arms of ecstasy.'

He slapped the Pol-47 — Police Form 47, which is filled out by the attending constable and contains all the relevant facts about the scene of death, the person and his or her life. It's usually on the strength of terse account contained in a Pol-47 that the coroner decides whether a post-mortem is required.

I picked it up.

'The deceased is 63 years old and has no medical history of note. He breakfasted this morning on porridge and saveloys, but refused the saveloys because he said they were hard and gristly.'

I sighed. Most Pol-47s contained these strangely irrelevant facts. What could you expect when they were taken by the most junior constable sent to the scene? If the family thought a piece of information was important, who was a young cop to judge?

I read on.

'He then left for work as usual. He is a salesman who travels to see a round of customers, selling hygienic merchandise to do with hand washing. A call was received at the Central Police Station at 11.30 hrs. The call was made by the owner of a local entertainment centre. The deceased appears to have succumbed while exercising, according to staff. There are no suspicious circumstances at the scene. His GP has been contacted and since he has not seen the deceased for three years is not prepared to sign the death certificate. The deceased man's car was legally parked down the road at a metered park. There was still 35 minutes to run on the meter.'

That is all there was. I looked up at Bruce, perplexed. 'I don't get it. So what on earth are the arms of ecstasy?'

Bruce rolled his eyes. 'Entertainment centre. It was a bloody knocking-shop, wasn't it? A whore-house. "Died while exercising", my arse!'

Bruce was right. There was always a trickle of males who had passed away in the act of intercourse, usually legitimately with their wives, but surprisingly often while with a prostitute. I supposed it was the high blood pressure that went with the heightened excitement that did it. Death in the arms of ecstasy. Some men might joke that it is a desirable way to go, but it could lead to major complications if they end up unexpectedly dead in the wrong place and in the wrong bed.

I knew what to look for, so the autopsy was brief. The answer, as expected, was in the coronary arteries, the only blood supply to the heart. I found a 60 per cent occlusion of the left coronary artery and a 90 per cent occlusion of the left anterior descending artery, the usual source of lethal heart attacks. There was a smidgen of haemorrhage underneath a fatty plaque in the artery. In his excitement, he had bled into one of the lesions in his artery. A bit of bleeding was all it took to close off the badly blocked artery completely.

I had seen it several times before. It was a pity, because he wasn't overweight, wasn't a diabetic and the blockage was quite localized. If it had been picked up earlier — yesterday morning, say — he could have had surgery. With a coronary artery bypass or a stent inserted across the fatty plaque, he might have lived for a while yet.

When I got back to my office, there was an invitation from Doug Brew to come up to the police station at six o'clock for drinks. There was a bar upstairs where the CIB members could relax and socialise without being out in the public eye. I accepted with pleasure, and settled down to write my preliminary opinion on the deceased's cause of death for the coroner. Graham Hubbard, the Palmerston North coroner, liked to have an advance note so he could have a chat with the family and tell them what had happened before his finding was handed down at the inquest.

Barely a quarter of an hour later, the hospital receptionist called to say there was a policeman wanting to see me. I was surprised. We had a hospital policeman who often came to see me with information, requests or more often just to gossip about what was happening around the hospital and in the Manawatu. He was a font of information and I usually knew what cases were likely to come my way even before the coroner had been informed. This couldn't be that man.

I went down to reception. A young constable stood there waiting, apparently ill at ease. He introduced himself and asked if I was the pathologist who performed the autopsy on the deceased we'd received that day. He was the officer sent to investigate the scene and had written the brief Pol-47 report. He wanted to have a private word with me. I was intrigued. This was unusual, and I was pretty sure it wasn't about the gristly saveloys.

I invited him up to the lab, where we could talk. No sooner had we got into my office than he thrust his hand into his pocket and pulled out an envelope. He didn't hand it to me, but placed it carefully on my desk and asked me to add it to the dead man's personal effects.

I opened it. There was $120 in it, a lot of money back then. I looked up at him, puzzled.

The constable looked embarrassed. He was perspiring lightly.

'It's the money that the deceased gentleman paid the, er, woman. You know, at the brothel. Apparently clients have to pay in advance. I felt that as the deceased hadn't finished, the woman had no right to the money. I found the woman in question and recovered the money from her. By rights, it should go back to the family.'

I must have looked as astonished as I felt. The young man looked at me defiantly.

'She wanted to argue the point with me,' he said. 'I had to be very firm with her before she would hand it over.'

'Don't you think she was doing everything she had contracted to do?' I asked gently. 'The way things turned out was more of an act of God than any fault of hers. Why should she return the money?'

He flushed brick red, but he was adamant. I could see the determination on his face. He was determined that the money must go back to the deceased's family.

There was nothing for it. I picked up the envelope and agreed to make sure it went to the right place. The constable look relieved. I suspect he might have been wondering if he had gone too far. He insisted on a receipt, which I improvised, scribbling on a piece of notepaper. He wanted me to count the money, but I declined, telling him I trusted him and with that he would have to leave it at that.

He shoved the receipt into his pocket, dumped his cap on his head and left as fast as he decently could.

In the Arms of Ecstasy

* * *

By quarter past six, I was comfortably ensconced in the police bar, a glass of whisky in my hand. The bar was warm and filled with the usual fug of smoke. Two hours and a couple of whiskies later, I felt light and comfortable. I could relax here. That is what the whisky was telling me.

I found myself telling them about the 'arms of ecstasy' and the problem I was having with the $120. They roared with laughter. A detective told me that his first homicide investigation had been at a brothel in Wellington. The client had refused to pay and the girl took to him with a short-handled spade, an entrenching tool from the First War. She apparently got off very lightly, all things considered. Opinion was that the judge quite liked the look of her and admired her spirited defence.

'So what are you going to do with the money?' someone asked.

'Oh, I think I'll find the woman and give it back,' I replied. I think I surprised them. I definitely surprised myself.

'You could compromise yourself,' someone mused. 'Better not. Wouldn't do for someone in your position to be seen handing over money to a working girl.'

'That's right,' another added. 'Lots of them are mixed up in gangs and that sort of stuff. Some of them are on drugs. You don't want to get tangled up in that kind of shit.'

I considered the advice. It made sense, sort of. Any thought of getting the police to return the money was out of the question, for precisely the reasons they'd offered.

'How would I find her, if I wanted to do it anyway?' I asked.

They all shrugged.

It's funny, but before the first whisky, I had no idea what I was going to do with the money. By the time I'd had a third whisky, I had more or less made up my mind to return it to the prostitute. The plan seemed right. Whisky is good like that.

By the next morning, as I laboured through my day examining specimens in the lab while nursing a serious headache, all thoughts of the money had gone out of my mind. It wasn't until I got back to my office and found a handwritten note on my desk with a name and an address, and an amount — $120 — that I remembered. The note was unsigned and I didn't recognise the writing. The lab receptionist hadn't seen anyone come through to my office, so I had no idea who had put it there. But I knew what it was about. Someone out there agreed with my plan of action and was helping me.

The address was just around the corner from where we lived. We were almost neighbours. I'm not sure why this was surprising. Sex workers have to live somewhere and someone is bound to be their neighbour. Why not us? I decided to return the money early that Saturday afternoon. After lunch, I played with our children, drawing it out. For the more I thought about my plan, the more ridiculous it seemed. I dithered even longer by deciding to mow the lawn, although it didn't really need doing. Displacement activity. It's what people usually do when they don't want to face up to something.

'Why don't you just put the envelope in her letterbox?' Elayne suggested.

'It's a lot of money to leave lying about,' I replied. 'How about you take it around?'

She stared at me as though I was mad.

I sighed. I knew I had to do it. I didn't even have any chores left to do.

I took my young daughter, Victoria, along as a chaperone. I even thought of taking our golden labrador, but decided against it, as there could be other dogs or cats there. The last thing I wanted was to create a scene.

I have to admit I was nervous. The woman's house was reasonably tidy, the garden neat, up to a point. But there was a lot of maintenance to be done. The spouting was obviously clogged with leaves and mould. I could see where the rain had spilled over and stained the stucco walls. I knocked on the door. My heart was racing. What a ridiculous situation to be in.

She wasn't what I expected. Actually, I wasn't sure who or what I'd been expecting. She wasn't tall and her dark hair was cut in a sort of pageboy style. She was pretty in an elfin way and wore glasses with thick frames. She was carrying a young boy, maybe a few months older than Vicky, on her hip.

'Hello?' she said. She smiled at Vicky, pushed her hair to one side and smiled interrogatively at me. Her voice was strangely gravelly.

'I've got something to give you,' I said. I shifted Vicky from one side to the other and pulled the now crumpled envelope from my pocket and passed it to her.

The Cause of Death

She took it uncertainly. She put her boy down and opened the envelope. For a moment she stared at the money and then looked back up at me, frowning, as I stood there holding Victoria.

'What's this for?' she asked.

I introduced myself and explained that I investigated deaths for the coroner. I told her where the money had come from. She blushed deeply as she realised what was happening.

She started talking rapidly. She told me her name and that the police officer had been rude, telling her that the death was entirely her fault and she was lucky she wasn't being charged.

I snorted. 'No. That's not right. He had no right to do that. The money's yours.'

She told me that the deceased was the first dead person she had ever seen. He'd turned black. As she spoke, her voice wobbled. It had obviously been an awful experience for her.

As soon as I decently could, I left. She walked with me to the gate.

'You should clear out your spouting,' I said, and pointed out where it had been overflowing.

She smiled. 'It's on my list. I've got to borrow a ladder from next door.'

She watched me strap Vicky into the car.

'Thank you,' she said. 'Thanks for doing that.'

I don't think she meant the spouting.

* * *

Late the next week, I had a call from reception saying they had something for me to collect.

I went down from my office to find a rather clumsily iced chocolate cake. It had been left by a young woman who wouldn't leave a name. There was a note with it.

'Thanks,' it read. There was nothing else, but I knew who had sent it.

I put the cake in the tearoom with a 'help yourself' note on it. I've never been a fan of chocolate cake.

CHAPTER 9

The Eggshell Skull

Usually it is the CIB who call the pathologist to a murder scene. We're given the story, the scene is described and the victim tentatively identified. We then gown up, and move slowly into the picture like a chameleon creeping along a branch. We have to step from foot-plate to foot-plate to avoid contaminating the scene. I swear the police get their tallest constable to set down the plates. The steps are often uncomfortably far apart, even for me, and I am quite tall.

Only once was I present at a murder scene before it had been properly designated as such, and before all the investigative protocols had been set in place. I'd been asked to look at an odd death that had puzzled the officers who had been called to the scene. The victim had been in hospital, had been unwell and had subsequently died at home. That alone made it seem unlikely there would be a problem. After all it's an occurrence that happens just about every day.

But the deceased was only 17 years old and there were some strange bloodstains present. I went to the house on Coventry Street in Highbury, a struggling part of town with a lot of cheap rentals and flats peopled by itinerant workers and beneficiaries. It was a known haunt of the gangs. Indeed, I was familiar with Coventry Street, because only a few weeks before, on Waitangi Day 2002, I had been called to the slaying of Black Power gang prospect Wallace Whatuira. He had been shot in the chest with a 12 gauge shotgun from close to point-blank range.

The scene of the Whatuira shooting was right next door to the one I was attending. This one was a simple rental, but looked quite tidy from the street. Some of the nearby yards were pretty shabby by comparison, with discarded bottles and rubbish scattered about.

The front door was ajar. A policeman came out to meet me. He pulled out his notebook and told me that the deceased person was Barbara Miller, female Caucasian, 17 years old. She had been in Palmerston North Hospital in the last week with paralysis of the arm and leg. She had been discharged with rehabilitation organised for follow-up.

That was an unusual story for starters. It sounded like a stroke, but she was very young for that

'Her partner, Basil Mist, phoned in this morning to say he'd found her dead in the hall,' the policeman went on. 'They were at a family dinner the night before and returned to the house about 9.30 p.m. He then went for a ride on his bike to visit a friend about midnight. He spent the night drinking with his friend and returned to find Barbara lying

The Cause of Death

in the hallway. He says he attempted resuscitation without success.'

The policeman confided that after listening to him, the police were sceptical about the resuscitation part of the story, because he couldn't tell them what it involved. He said he'd blown into her lungs and made downward jabs with his hands. The police doubted anyone had touched the body after she had collapsed.

* * *

The deceased was lying on her back in the hall, head against a wall radiator. She was a pretty girl, but painfully thin, tall with short, dark, ragged hair. She was wearing a simple dress, pale with some pastel designs, stained here and there with dried, ochre-coloured blood. The dress was hitched up around her waist. Her legs were apart and there was dried blood on them. This did not look like a natural death to me, despite the story of hospitalisation. In fact it looked suspiciously like a rape.

But if it were a sexual assault, there were oddities, and these had puzzled the police at the scene, too.

In her tightly clenched hand was a damp facecloth, also bloodstained but more heavily than her dress. Her mouth was gaping and I could see pale, cream-coloured vomit filling up her mouth right up to her incisor teeth. I found a small cut on the top of her scalp — the only injury — so the blood had come from there. It seemed likely she was holding the cloth to her scalp when — when what happened? Vomiting and inhalation of the vomit must have been the final event, but why? How did this relate to the paralysis to one side of her body? Could she have a brain tumour? Vomiting with a brain tumour was common.

It certainly looked suspicious. I had a look around.

There were bloodstains all along one side of the hall but they were trifling smears only. They were all at hand height and reminded me of the Junction Motel. There was quite a lot of blood in the bathroom and there were strands of her hair in the basin.

It looked as if she had received a cut to her head, gone to the bathroom to wash and get the facecloth, and then staggered along the hall, supporting herself on the wall with one hand. The other hand would be holding the cloth to her head wound, I would guess. Then, here at the front door, something happened and she fell over, vomited and died.

I thought hard. I couldn't think of any natural explanation. I shook my head and decided. This death must be treated as suspicious until matters became clearer.

The CIB team rapidly and professionally swung into action. Detective Senior Sergeant Craig Sheridan was in charge of the investigation. There was also a scene of crime officer, or SOCO, and a constable in change of the body, the OC Body.

There were pathology investigations that I needed to start right away in order to try to get an estimate of how long the victim had been dead. The sooner I could start, the more accurate the calculation would be.

The Cause of Death

As usual I was assigned a new, young constable to assist. I could see he was nervous. I suspected, though, that this might be his first murder and his first body.

First I examined her for *rigor mortis*, the stiffening of muscles to a state of rigidity that comes on in a predictable sequence after death. Her jaw was clenched rigidly. Her arms and legs, too, were stiff and unbendable. Finally I took her hand and gently tried to prise her fingers open, but they were like talons.

Rigor mortis was complete and involving all muscle groups, so I thought the body was as rigid as it was going to get. I would retest the muscles in two hours to see if there had been any change.

All muscles contract in death and become rigid. There are many variables, but generally the jaw muscles tighten first, followed by the arms, then legs and finally the small muscles of the hands. If you start early enough, you can record the sequence of changes and get an idea of when the process started. Unfortunately it was a dead-end here as the sequence was probably complete. All that told me was that she had died between 10 and 20 hours ago. That was a pretty wide window, but it was a start.

I gently rolled Barbara's body over. Her back was a deep and unnatural purple colour, mottled, with crease marks from her hitched up dress making a startling white zigzag across her lower back. The pattern from the threadbare pile of the hall carpet was also imprinted on her buttock.

'Christ. Is that bruising? the policeman asked.

'No, it's what we call lividity,' I replied. 'After death, the blood sinks to the lowest parts of the body. In this case, it's settled out in her back and buttocks because she was half-slumped against the wall.'

I pushed firmly with my thumb on the largest patch of lividity. After 30 seconds' pressure my white thumbprint remained on the skin. I nodded in satisfaction.

'The lividity blanches or disappears with prolonged pressure,' I told the cop. 'That means the settling out of the blood isn't complete. It takes around 12 hours after death.'

That gave me a first, rough estimate for the time of death of about 11 o'clock the previous night. I would keep checking until the lividity stopped spreading and no longer blanched. That would happen about 20 hours after death and might support my first time fix.

I went back into my bag and brought out a long thermometer, specially designed to measure temperatures accurately between 0 and 40 degrees centigrade. I also picked up a scalpel handle and carefully slid on a new blade.

'I'm going to measure the temperature of her body and the room,' I explained. 'I can look the temperatures up in a set of tables and get an estimated time of death.'

I held the thermometer about 30 centimetres above the body and measured the room temperature. Then I made a small incision in the stomach wall and slid the thermometer into the abdominal cavity. I spared the policeman the explanation. Pathologists usually take the body temperature either anally or vaginally, but that can interfere with DNA testing in rape cases. My first forensics teacher, Kevin Lee, had advised using the technique I was using now.

Once I finished recording the temperatures, I took out a syringe and fitted a needle.

'Hang on. This can be a bit of a shock,' I told the cop. I inserted the needle into the sclera — the tough, white outer coat — of one eyeball.

I drew out the vitreous humour, or eyeball fluid.

'What the fuck is that for?' the policeman asked in a strange, strangled voice.

'We measure the amount of potassium in the eye. We do other readings, but mainly potassium. When you're alive, the potassium in the eye is very low, but it gradually increases at a reasonably uniform rate after death. There are ways to calculate an estimated time of death from the potassium levels.'

'Right,' he said. 'Nice.'

I would come back in two hours to repeat all these tests in order to detect any changes and collect the fluid from the other eye. Then I would recalculate so that I had two readings to compare. Hopefully they would support each other.

No one method was fool-proof, which is why you try to perform the whole range. All are subject to many variables, and of course, defence lawyers know each and every one and were experts at demolishing the evidence. Their technique is to cut down the evidence, tree by tree, and then say: 'You see? There never was a wood here, was there?'

* * *

As I performed my tests, the team at the house were working hard. Every detail was painstakingly recorded. A photographer was recording the blood smears on the wall. With repeated flashes he captured the imprints from every conceivable angle. He also took preliminary photographs of the body and asked if there were anything in particular we wanted shots of. I thought a close-up of the vomit in the mouth, because that was unusual and I didn't know off-hand how that came to be. Most people when vomiting hurl it out, but that hadn't happened here. Why not?

We gathered outside the house so that I could present my early results, which can be critical in helping focus the direction of the investigation.

All I was able to contribute at this stage was that the cause of death seemed to be inhalation of vomit. There was a relatively small cut on the top of the head, and while this was probably not directly relevant to death, it was evidence of an assault. I thought an assault more likely than an accidental injury as it was right on the top of the head. I couldn't think of an obvious way to get such an injury accidentally. It was more likely to have been sustained from a blow from above.

I was asked about rape. At first glance, it seemed possible, but I thought she was probably dead upon hitting the ground. I wasn't really sure why. It was just a feeling. Of course a rape can also occur after death: the post-mortem would tell us whether that had happened.

Even at this early stage, I was able to give an estimate for the time of death. In the victim's case, the calculations were all giving a similar answer, which increased my confidence. My estimate was between 10.30 and 11 the previous night — plus or minus several hours, of course. I would have to report the range of variation and uncertainty. But I was confident the index time was about right.

'That's helpful,' DSS Sheridan said. 'We've got young Basil Mist down at the station giving a statement. He's not very happy at the moment. He's being seriously abusive to the interrogating officers. We'll be questioning him up for a while until we're happy with what he's saying. Could be quite a while if he's still being a shit-stirrer and telling us to fuck off. We'll just have to see. We anticipate moving the body to the mortuary by late afternoon. When can you do the post-mortem?'

'I think I'll do it tonight. That'll pretty well exclude any obvious natural causes and then we'll know whether to carry on or can it. Besides, tomorrow's pretty busy for me at the hospital so I'd like to get it over with now, if possible.'

I managed to report out a dozen biopsies and then went home for an early dinner.

* * *

By 9 p.m. we were ready to start the post-mortem. Bruce and I were at the table where the victim was laid out and there was a full complement of detectives seated in the gallery.

'Look at this, Doctor.' Bruce's face was sorrowful. He pointed at the victim's head.

The hair was crawling with *Pediculosis capitis*, the head louse. As the body cooled in the fridge waiting for me, the headlice had awoken and were off in search of a warmer host. We often saw that in the mortuary, particularly in younger people. Head lice were a sign of poverty, of helplessness. Most of our families have had the odd infestation, but we have the knowledge and resources to get rid of them. This poor young waif had no hope. She weighed only 41 kilograms and her body was covered with 45 different bruises, abrasions and scratches. Her ribs had been repeatedly fractured — the tragic diary of poverty, repeated assaults and abuse over a long period of time.

I began my examination. The airway was crammed full of vomit, as I had suspected. This was clearly what had killed her. I opened the gullet into the stomach. The stomach was very full. The food had been churned into a creamy chyme, the same vomit that I had found blocking the airway from the teeth to the lungs. There was about a litre and a half of the stuff. None of it was recognisable, although there were a few threads that I thought might be rhubarb, or possibly celery. The same material was also in the duodenum.

'This is very interesting.'

The detectives, tired and hungry from the long hours they were putting in on this investigation, looked up.

'The stomach is still full with only a small amount of semi-digested food in the duodenum. In a normal person, that would be the case roughly one to two hours after eating. Do you know when she ate the family meal? That could give us another marker as to the time of death. It's an unreliable measure, especially as she's been sick recently and her stomach may not be functioning normally, but it could be worth doing.'

DSS Sheridan nodded.

The Cause of Death

'We'll get someone onto the timings tomorrow.'

The scalp wound was small, as I had already observed, no more than a centimetre in length, with cleanly slit edges as if made by a knife. There was a curious, patterned indentation on the surface of the skull bone. The bone was indented over five millimetres by six tightly spaced, parallel grooves. They were obviously an imprint from the weapon that had caused the wound and there was no doubt that significant force was used in order to dent the skull bone. But what sort of weapon might make such a pattern? And was it accidental or intentional? Whatever the weapon, the pattern was quite distinctive and we ought to be able to identify the weapon exactly.

It wasn't until some days later that I hit upon the answer to the ridged dents grooved into the skull. Like most things, once you've recognised it, you wonder why you didn't see it before. By sheer chance, I happened to tap on a block of butter with the serrated tip of a dinner knife. I looked down in surprise at exactly the pattern seen on poor Barbara's skull. The weapon was a dinner knife, one with a finely milled and serrated tip that had been brought down violently in a stabbing motion onto the top of the victim's head. The size of the wound fitted a dinner knife as the weapon and so did the injury on the bone.

Otherwise there was nothing remarkable in the autopsy: no evidence of a rape, no natural cause of death. The cause of death was a mystery until I lifted the brain out of the skull and began to dissect it. There was no tumour, as I had wondered. But the brain was far from normal. There were

The Eggshell Skull

a number of strange, brownish discolourations scattered through the white matter of the brain and these stained the critical nerve transmission pathways.

What on earth was this? It was certainly pathological, but what was it and how did it relate to the extraordinary circumstances in which the victim had been found?

I described what I was seeing but I had to tell Craig and his CIB team that I was not sure what it meant.

'So, are you saying that she may have a medical disease? That this might not be murder at all?'

'It's possible,' I admitted. 'I'm really sorry that I can't be more definite at this stage. What I can say is that her brain is distinctly abnormal. That fits with her being in hospital before with hemiplegia, a paralytic stroke. But this obviously just doesn't add up with what we found at the scene.'

'When will you know?'

'Realistically, three days to process the tissue, make slides and diagnose them.'

'Three days. That long?' Craig looked thoughtful. 'We'll have to treat this as a homicide until you tell us otherwise. If we don't, we may lose valuable time that we'll never get back. We'll continue the investigation. We'll meet at 0800 tomorrow in the briefing room at the station to assign tasks. And now, if we're finished, I suggest everybody gets away for some food and sleep. I have a feeling that this may become quite big.'

I had the same feeling.

* * *

The Cause of Death

I examined the victim's brain tissue under the microscope the next morning. It was puzzling. There were white cells — macrophages filled with fat — engulfing the lipid-rich brain tissue. But I knew these cells took at least five days in living tissue before they came to look like this. So clearly I was looking at a disease that preceded her death by at least that much.

This finding just did not support murder. What was happening here?

I sat back and thought. I could find no inspiration, but my instincts told me this wasn't right. Something bad had happened here. I needed help, professionally at least. So I sent the victim's brain slides to a neuropathologist for another opinion. Until that returned I could not advance the diagnosis.

Craig called me often, pushing for an answer. I think the more they looked at Basil Mist, the less they liked him. A detective said to me: 'He's a particularly bad bit of work if ever I've seen one.' I sensed they knew more than they were letting on, but they would need concrete evidence if they were to charge and detain him.

The only thing I could state with a reasonable degree of confidence was that my estimate of the time of death was confirmed, so far as science could determine. The time of 11 p.m. the night before we examined the body still looked about right to me.

* * *

It was early on Monday morning and I had just settled down to diagnose my routine cases when my phone rang. The police were here already. They really needed an answer, but I didn't have one yet.

Apparently Basil had arrived on the scene some years before, when Barbara was a very young and vulnerable teenager. They started a relationship and Basil moved into an abandoned car lying in the back of the family yard. The neighbours were shocked at the going-on. Barbara had had two daughters by Basil over the years. He was fierce, physical and highly aggressive and everyone in Barbara's family lived in terror of him. His relationship with Barbara was extremely violent, but neither she nor anyone else felt they could do anything about it. There were regular beatings taking place even in front of her mother, who was powerless to stop it. Basil moved into the family home and began to take it over.

Basil dragged Barbara off to live in Coventry Street in Highbury, from where he continued his reign of terror over the family from a distance. At this point, Barbara was taken ill and taken to the hospital. There she was found to be paralysed down one side of her body.

I knew this part already. I had checked out her medical records from the hospital. According to the records, she presented with paralysis of the left arm and leg — basically a hemiplegia — as well as some suspicious bruises that she couldn't explain. The house surgeon's note speculated that it was the result of an assault, but she denied it. They didn't pursue the issue. The diagnosis was a moderately dense hemiplegia with some loss of sensation. No cause for this was found, and as she began to show signs of rapid recovery, it was thought that the cause was functional, which is to say,

The Cause of Death

they felt her symptoms were due to psychological reasons rather than to an underlying organic disease. It was in her mind, not in her brain. In war, many soldiers develop odd forms of paralysis after being shelled: shell-shock, neurasthenia, post-traumatic stress disorder ... There are lots of complicated names but we have little insight into the cause and mechanism. We just don't know enough about the way the mind works.

Of course, the physicians knew that Barbara was in an abusive relationship and was quite young, both of which are common backgrounds for functional brain disorders.

Detective Senior Sergeant Craig Sheridan wanted to know if any of this had a bearing on what I had found. Did it establish a cause of death that the police could work with?

I had to admit that I was no further ahead on that, although I could say that the physician who diagnosed a functional paralysis was quite wrong. The changes I had found in the brain showed, beyond doubt, that there was evidence of an underlying disease. But I didn't yet know what the disease was, or how it related to Barbara's paralysis, or what it had to do with the manner of her death.

But Craig had gleaned a curious piece of further information from Barbara's mother. Oddly enough, Barbara had two younger brothers, both of whom died in strange circumstances at school. Two? That definitely was not normal. And her mother suffered a cardiac arrest herself on witnessing her second son's collapse.

'What were the circumstances of the brothers' deaths?' I asked.

'Apparently one drowned in front of a number of people while in a swimming pool. The other had a number of seizures and died while playing in a park and climbing a rugby post.' Craig shook his head sadly. 'Poor woman had to go through that, and now her daughter is dead as well.'

'But this is extraordinary. What on earth could have happened? How can two boys die unexpectedly and so publicly, for God's sake? That can't be right. They must have had an underlying medical problem surely? But what is it?'

I knew this must be important and that the siblings' deaths must be linked in some mysterious way. I had this niggling thought about familial epilepsy. It is very rare but I wondered if it was the unrecognised disease that was killing this family. And of course, there was something pathologically abnormal in the victim's brain. That needed to be diagnosed before we could dispel the fog of confusion in which we laboured.

'I'll get out their autopsy reports and have a look into it,' I told Craig.

'Weren't you going to send the slides for an expert opinion?'

'Yes, I've done that. They've been posted to Beth Synec, a neuropathologist in Auckland. But I won't hear anything for at least another fortnight or so.'

'A fortnight? Oh, shit.'

* * *

Getting back to work, I pulled my neuropathology textbook from my bookcase and looked up familial epilepsy. There were only two lines of text and the second was intriguing. I read: 'One case report documents two siblings both of whom are considered to have died from SUDEP.' Sudden Unexpected Death in Epilepsy. Could this be it?

I found a reference that mentioned Professor Sam Berkovic at the University of Melbourne. I decided to collect all the information from the brothers' medical records and post-mortem reports, as well as my findings from Barbara's, and send it all off to him and ask whether he thought this might be a case of familial epilepsy.

I had no problem finding the brothers' post-mortem reports, which were filed in the gloomy, dusty basement beneath the hospital. There were even the histological slides and tissues taken from the boys at autopsy for examination. Alas, there was not much to find. All the tissue sections were normal and the police report in both cases had little to add to what had previously been outlined to me.

What's more, in both cases, the pathologist had considered that the cause of death was natural. A coroner had agreed. But it still seemed impossible to me that two healthy boys had both died unexpectedly in the flush of their youth without there being some common factor. And how were their deaths relevant to Barbara?

* * *

I was right: it was exactly two weeks later that I heard from Beth Synec.

The Eggshell Skull

I called Craig at once and read the contents of the letter to him.

'The lesions are most likely to have occurred following the blockage of small blood vessels by small blood clots travelling to the brain. This may include episodes of an irregular heartbeat, during which tiny clots may form in the heart, perhaps between muscle bundles. Later these may be thrown off and travel to the brain. The strokes were about three weeks old, fitting precisely with the victim's onset of paralysis and admission to hospital. They were on both sides of the brain so must have come from the heart or aorta.'

Included in her letter was more highly technical information and evidence, but that was the gist of it.

'Thank you for sharing this case with me,' she concluded. 'I would be interested to hear the outcome in due course.'

'Emboli are clots carried to the brain in the blood,' I went on to explain to Craig. 'They destroy the brain tissue by blocking the arteries. But where did the emboli come from? It can only be from the heart, it just has to be, but that was entirely normal at autopsy.'

'So it's a natural death, then?' He sounded disappointed.

'On the face of it, yes, but the facts just don't tie up. How does it fit with the head injury and what about the strange scene of death? None of that part can possibly be natural, never mind what was in the brain.'

But there was more odd evidence. That is always the way. TV programmes like *CSI* seem so clean and crisp but in reality murder investigations are often confusing, with too much irrelevant information. Those involved have to winnow the chaff away to find the kernels of truth.

A check of Basil's cell phone showed multiple calls made in rapid succession soon after the couple arrived home, but these stopped abruptly. The activity occurred squarely across my estimated time of death.

'Do you know what the calls were about?' I asked.

'Well, as a matter of fact, we do. Apparently it's something kids do these days. There's a theory going around that if you dial the number of a large company repeatedly, then somehow you can break into their network. You can use this trick to dial up 0900 numbers and listen to pornography for free. It's actually a myth, but apparently a lot of kids spend quite a bit of time trying.'

It was another week until the darkness finally began to lift. It started with a reply from Professor Sam Berkovic in Melbourne, answering my questions.

'I know of no specific form of familial epilepsy that has a high propensity for sudden death. Indeed, most familial epilepsies are relatively mild and the tragic story of this family would be extraordinary and certainly out of the realm of experience that I am aware of personally and from the literature. I therefore think the diagnosis of familial epilepsy is quite unlikely.

'I think there is positive evidence though that this family had a familial arrhythmia, presumably a long QT syndrome.'

The QT syndrome was new to me. Twenty minutes later, I was on the phone to Dr Jon Skinner, a paediatric cardiologist at Greenlane Hospital who headed the Cardiac

Inherited Disease Registry. He had been on a mission to have significant cardiac deaths in young New Zealand adults investigated for the prolonged QT gene mutations.

'Yes, yes,' he said enthusiastically after I told him the story. 'This certainly sounds like a case of a prolonged QT syndrome.'

He explained how microscopic channels in the heart carried and regulated sodium and potassium and kept the electrical environment of the heart stable. An abnormality in these channels could give rise to a variety of symptoms, from a racing heart to fainting and even sudden death. I learned how there were seven types. Type 1 typically causes sudden death in athletes, particularly when swimming.

Here, finally, was the breakthrough we'd been looking for. This might be what had happened to Barbara's brothers.

'There's an oddity here,' cautioned Dr Skinner. 'The boys sound like Type 1 but the Type 2 is a better fit for the mother's collapse and, of course, that of your victim, Barbara. You see, in the Type 2, sudden death is brought on by emotional stress or getting a fright. We have heard of cases where it has even been brought on by an alarm clock going off and for others by a telephone call at night while asleep. There are even stories about crying babies precipitating these attacks.'

'What must I do to prove a QT syndrome? This would be critical evidence if there is a court case.'

'I'll need to see and examine the girl's mother and father as well as any surviving brothers and sisters. We need to find if there are any existing ECGs in any of the victim's hospital records. That will tell us whether they had prolonged QT intervals, although these may not necessarily be present at all times in the ECG traces. If I can prove the disease in the family, then you can argue strongly that your dead girl had it, too.'

'That would be helpful, but in a court of law it may not be enough unless we can *prove* that Barbara had it too. Is that possible?'

There was a long silence. It had never been done on post-mortem tissue before but he agreed to try to find the mutation. I felt the answer was getting closer.

* * *

My working theory was that Basil assaulted Barbara with a blow to the head and the intense emotion and fear caused an irregular heartbeat. Then, because her heart was beating irregularly, the blood flow in one of the chambers was disturbed and formed a clot. That happens quite commonly, and bits of the clot can then break off and go to the brain, causing a stroke.

The flaw in the argument was that the brain changes were ten days old. How did that fit with the attack on her that night? Perhaps these were two separate but similar events. An irregular heartbeat ten days before was precipitated by something else. Another assault was possible given the bruises seen when she was in hospital. Maybe that is what caused the paralysis and the admission to hospital the first time a week before. The attack with the dinner knife on the night on the death was another event. That attack would have precipitated

The Eggshell Skull

a second arrhythmia and that's what led to Barbara's death. If it was true that she had a prolonged QT syndrome, then she would be a sitting duck for any number of attacks at later times with many different precipitating causes, some of them potentially quite trivial. But surely that would mean that death could be attributed to natural causes. How could this be murder?

* * *

'The Crown Prosecutor is on the line, Doctor.'

I had just arrived in my office. It was Ben Vanderkolk.

'Can I talk to you this morning? It's about the Barbara Miller case. There is an important development.'

I was shown into Ben's office shortly after 10 a.m.

'Thanks so much for coming at such short notice.'

We sat down. I explained where my investigation had led.

'This is complex and we're only just getting to the bottom of it now.' I outlined my findings and how I had laboriously put together what they meant. 'So my best theory is that Barbara, and her deceased brothers, all have a prolonged QT syndrome. The most likely scenario is that final night she was so frightened and emotionally agitated by the attack that it precipitated a final arrhythmia. During the attack she vomited, inhaled the vomit and died.'

Ben looked at me questioningly, deep in concentration. There was a silence.

'And there is no doubt that the injuries that she suffered during the assault were relatively minor and did not directly cause her death, but yet could or would have caused the fatal arrhythmia?'

I nodded. 'Yes. That's exactly it. That's what I think happened.'

'Very, very interesting,' he murmured. 'Yes. This is a great outcome. Yes, it will do perfectly.'

'How can this be a great outcome? Surely it argues that the immediate cause of death was natural?'

'It's the "Eggshell Skull" argument. It's well recognised in law and I've always wanted to argue this particular principle in court. It goes like this. If you hit somebody on the head lightly and you kill them because they happen to be born with a fragile skull, then you're still responsible for their death. The law believes that you take your victim as you find them, whether they might have an eggshell skull or not, and you're therefore still responsible for the consequences of your actions, no matter what.'

He smiled as something else occurred to him.

'What makes it worse for Basil is that he had assaulted her ten days before and that caused her paralysis then. So he knew that even a minor assault could have serious consequences. I will therefore charge Basil with murder, and run a prosecution based on the thin eggshell skull precedent. This is going to be a landmark case. I believe there's enough evidence and I'll get the conviction. Of that I am absolutely certain.'

* * *

'The Law grinds slowly but surely,' is the old saying. When it's ready, it's ready. It was to be nearly a year later before I was called to court.

Sometimes murders that happened years apart were heard within days of each other, making for huge differences in testing of evidence, availability of lawyers, judges and a host of factors. I personally found this a challenge because I had to put myself back into scenes that had happened long ago. And believe me, a person's views and degree of tolerance can and do change from day to day. A story that might just be believable on one day might be quite preposterous the next. A jury might convict on the evidence on Monday but not on Thursday. Neither was wrong. We are humans and our foibles are the best the law can deliver.

I had reviewed all the facts of the case and felt prepared, not only to give evidence before the jury, but also for a briefing session with the public prosecutor to make sure that all the evidence and its place and strength was completely understood. I was also available to meet with the defence lawyers to explain the findings, hear and consider any alternative explanations they may have. It's important to keep an open mind. On occasions, the scenario painted by the defence lawyers on behalf of their clients has served to change my views, or at least modify them.

'Yes,' I might say, 'your explanation of events is certainly possible. The one I have outlined to the Crown is also possible but I cannot in all honesty weigh one as more likely than the other on purely scientific grounds.'

And then it would be up to the jury to decide which explanation they believed.

It was here in court that all the hard work by the police and, of course, my own work come together. The fine threads of evidence are woven into ever thicker cords until finally the strong rope of justice is fashioned. The accused has their say. Experts are called in by the defence to examine the evidence, including my autopsy evidence, for its strength and to seek out and expose any vulnerability.

I had gone over the thick dossier of photographs taken at the murder scene and autopsy. I had spent many hours going through the findings and now knew as much as anyone about cardiac arrhythmias, the prolonged QT syndrome and its sudden and tragic manifestations.

I scrutinised every photograph closely, checking there were explanations for everything. This had to be done carefully for that same volume of photographs and every piece of evidence was currently sitting on Mike Behrens' desk. Mike was an outstanding lawyer and he was acting for Basil Mist. He would be as diligent in searching for weaknesses in the Crown's case as Ben Vanderkolk would be to make sure it was watertight.

Jon Skinner's Auckland laboratory had done their best, but frustratingly was unable to demonstrate the abnormal gene for the QT disorder in Barbara's post-mortem tissues. Maybe tissue from the dead needed a different technique. No-one knew for sure.

I didn't think this negative result would influence the jury. The genetic studies were still very new and had been pretty much hit and miss up to that date. It was known that the studies did not identify all affected patients. No doubt there were other mutations yet to be discovered.

I was surprised to hear that there was more to come out about Basil Mist and his past.

After watching his behaviour, the police were sure that he was a bad one. His arrest brought a number of cases to a head. He had agreed to give a DNA sample and that broke a log-jam.

Basil was a serial rapist and the police had been searching for him for some time. His mode of operation was to use extreme violence and unlike most rapists, who use condoms, he was quite careless about leaving his semen behind. I expect Basil knew little or nothing about DNA testing. He would later be convicted of raping a 12-year-old girl at knifepoint in the Esplanade Gardens in Palmerston North, sexually violating a seven- and a 14-year-old girl, and of two further charges of sex with underage girls.

I was appalled. Of course, none of this could be revealed to the jury during the murder trial. It seemed to me logical that the pattern of his behaviour was absolutely relevant for a jury to know, but the law said that Basil could only be tried for one crime or set of related crimes at a time. Each trial needs a new jury and they aren't allowed to know anything about the person's previous crimes or any pending future charges.

* * *

Basil Mist, the killer of the fragile Barbara, was charged with Barbara's murder, found guilty of manslaughter and sentenced to open-ended preventative detention. The 'eggshell skull' argument had won the day. The sentence was overturned on appeal in view of his youth and a 20-year prison term substituted. He has not yet achieved parole and won't be eligible for release until January 2023.

Jon Skinner's tireless lobbying for the follow-up of unexpected cardiac deaths has borne fruit. All pathologists are now familiar with prolonged QT syndrome and arrange for testing for this gene mutation when it seems relevant. The legacy of the dead to their families in these cases is immense. They are usually active young people who die on the sports fields or when exercising, much to the immense shock and sorrow of their families. When their genes are also found in surviving family members, they can have artificial cardiac defibrillators inserted and be started on stabilising drugs to prevent sudden death. Their outlook is thought to be favourable. In that sense, the death of Barbara and others like her should never be thought of as in vain. Their deaths, if properly investigated, will provide a legacy of life to their families.

CHAPTER 10

Trouble with the Babysitter

'See for yourself,' Bruce Lockett said.

The answers to complex forensic problems sometimes take years or even decades for the truth to emerge. The specimen that Bruce had invited me to examine had been collected two years previously. It was the lung tissue of Samantha Rei Wales, who had been eight months old at the time of her death in the winter of 1991. In the absence of any evidence to the contrary, we had advised the coroner that this was a case of SUDI (sudden death in infancy, or 'cot death', to give it its common name).

The aspect of her case that was troubling was that she had been under the care of a babysitter when she died. At the time, I had felt terribly sorry for Heather Ross, the babysitter. What a horrific position to find yourself in, I thought. I deeply admired the Wales family for standing by Ross, their friend and neighbour, after Samantha's death. The family even allowed her to look after their remaining child, against the advice of the paediatrician. Although there were no suspicious circumstances, I wasn't sure I could have done the same.

Now, two years on, we were re-examining Samantha's lung tissue, because her sister Emma had been found dead, apparently of cot death, also while in Heather Ross's charge. And while I hadn't been able to detect anything awry on first examination, a fluke had turned our assumptions on their head.

I bent to the microscope. The view was like that through a kaleidoscope, a patchwork of pinks and intense blues.

'Good God,' I said. 'You're right. It's the same.'

'I've sent the samples to David Becroft,' Bruce said. 'Hopefully he can tell us what it means.'

'How the hell did you come to stain for iron in the first place?' I asked. 'It's hardly a routine test.'

Bruce shrugged. 'Serendipity.' He smiled. 'I saw some pigment which I thought might be iron in the slide of the liver and spleen and decided to test it. But I accidentally gave the wrong slide number to the technologists. They did the Perls stain on the lung slide instead. As soon as I saw it, I realised we had something significant here.'

Serendipity — stumbling across something by fortunate chance — has so often been the saviour of science.

The Perls test involves staining a tissue sample with a dye that reacts with iron compounds to produce an intense blue. The blue blaze on the slide I was looking at indicated that the cells lining the lung — in the macrophages and encrusted on the alveolar walls — were studded with iron.

I had never seen such heavy deposits of iron outside very rare cases shown at conferences.

This was Samantha's slide. We had only come to perform the Perls test on this one after Bruce Lockett had made his serendipitous discovery on Emma's tissue. Both exhibited the striking, anomalous iron deposits. We had kicked around the possibilities of which we were aware. There was, for example, a condition known as pulmonary haemosiderosis, which was rare but not unknown in children. As we read up about it, we found that pulmonary haemosiderosis can occur due to an allergy to cow's milk in children. It's a rare disease called Heiner syndrome. The other distinct possibility was a fungal infection. There were reports that heavy infections of toxic moulds were often found in the damp homes of children with pulmonary haemosiderosis.

We felt we didn't have the expertise to make a pronouncement, so we had dispatched the slides to David Becroft, a highly respected pathologist with a lifetime's expertise in paediatric pathology. He turned his agile mind to the question of how the iron deposits might have happened. Could it be pulmonary haemosiderosis?

His determination, when it came back, was stunning. He considered pulmonary haemosiderosis to be unlikely. He pointed out that deposits of iron in the lungs were very rare and quite limited in the usual cases of cot death, but were strongly positive and widely distributed in cases where children were known to have been serially suffocated. He felt that what we were seeing on the lungs of both dead girls was evidence of repeated attempts to smother them.

(Drs Becroft and Lockett later published their findings and were internationally recognised for their superb deduction. Thanks to them, performing a Perls stain on lung tissue is now regarded as a very important test to prove these cases.)

Meanwhile, the Wales had an anonymous, late-night call saying it was the girls' mother, Sherilyn, who had killed the children. Both believed they recognised the voice. It was Heather Ross. And there was more. A note was put in their letterbox, composed of letters crudely clipped from a variety of magazines and newspapers. It reminded me of the notes from the Brent Garner case. The content was the heavy stuff you'd expect. It must have been terrible for the Wales to have to deal with this business on top of losing their second daughter. God knows what kind of guilt they must be feeling. They confirmed that Dr Malcolm, their paediatrician, had told them never to use Heather Ross to babysit again.

The police were out on a scent again, but like the Wales, and despite the mounting evidence, I found it almost impossible to believe Heather Ross could be responsible. Why would she do this?

A police psychologist was able to put forward a theory.

'It could be Munchausen Syndrome by Proxy,' he said.

'What?' I had heard of Munchausen's Syndrome, of course, but I had never heard of this version.

'It's usually done by a mother to her own children,' he explained. 'The mother either invents or causes symptoms in her children, sometimes actually harming them. Apparently they want the attention and sympathy that they get from others because of their child's alleged disease. I've never come across a case. But this could be something like it. Perhaps the babysitter was doing it to get attention for herself?'

It all fitted, especially with the GP's reports of Emma's presentation with apnoeic episodes that she only ever suffered when she was in Ross's care. Then there was the deranged phone call, and the poison pen letter …

The trial of Heather Sylvie Ross on two counts of manslaughter eventually came before the court. The jury listened to the evidence with great concentration and with more than a tinge of sadness. When their verdict was handed down — Ross was found guilty on both counts of manslaughter — the jury looked very sombre. We all felt it. We had now glimpsed a very strange and disturbing side of our humanity. She was sentenced to nine years' imprisonment.

I regretted our failure to detect that something was seriously amiss two years before, when Samantha had died. I just wish we'd all looked harder or thought differently back then; maybe that would have changed the outcome. But it wasn't to be. What we have learned from Samantha's and Emma's deaths is that we must investigate all cot deaths thoroughly even though it is a difficult task at an emotional time. As Detective Sergeant Ross Grantham, who led the investigation, aptly said: 'It is an area of broken glass we have to walk over.'

* * *

We all love weekends. The cares of the week are behind us, the unsolved problems are shelved for the moment and we can return to work on Monday ready to confront the new problems that will surely arise. Like many of us I had so little time for my family during the week that I always looked forward to Saturday and my weekend time with them.

The great advantage of being a pathologist is the weekends are free of the long hours of caring for patients that so exhausted my clinical colleagues. So other than the rare event of a murder or suspicious death we could count on being free to wander and play all day through the tranquil beauty of the New Zealand countryside.

We were packed up one Sunday, Elayne held the picnic basket, the children were ready and Shumba was tearing around in anticipation, scattering the discarded Sunday newspaper lying on the floor. I took one last look around to make sure that I had everything we needed. Yes it was all there, the stove was off and we were away. As I locked the door the phone rang.

I hesitated. What could this be? I heard the police were tramping somewhere up in the Ruahine Ranges, following up a report from a pig hunter who'd found a pile of bones in the bush and thought they might be human. So it might be about that.

I unlocked the door and answered the phone.

'Hello, is that Dr Temple-Camp? Graham Hubbard, Coroner for Palmerston North here.'

'Yes, speaking, Mr Hubbard.' My heart was sinking fast. A call from the coroner was never good news for pathologists. Not as bad as a call from the police of course, because that inevitably meant a murder, which would tie me up for many days. But the coroner was bad enough. It surely meant something terrible had happened.

'I'm sorry to call you on a Sunday, but I have just been advised of a tragedy and I would like your help if possible.'

'Yes, of course. What has happened?'

'There has been a cot death in Woodville.'

Cot deaths had been a dreadful epidemic throughout the country prior to the early 1990s. Too many shocked parents had awoken to find a cold and blue baby in the morning. Despite a huge amount of investigation and meticulous autopsies no common thread had been found for decades. Certainly some of these babies showed minor signs of a lung infection. Rarely did we discover clear abnormalities that might have caused their death.

It had been a big mystery until Dr Shirley Tonkin in Auckland had made a major breakthrough. After a careful study of the anatomy of the throat and airway of an infant, she deduced that putting babies face downwards would make them vulnerable to suffocation, particularly if they had a minor cold and some swelling of the upper air passages. The incorrect advice given for so many years to put babies to sleep face downward was reversed in a nationwide campaign during the mid-90s.

It worked.

There was a dramatic fall in the number of cot deaths. We pathologists certainly noticed with relief how few new cot deaths we were receiving in the mortuary. But we still saw them, now and then. And they still needed an investigation in our search for answers.

The Cause of Death

'Normally I wouldn't trouble you until Monday morning. But there are some exceptional circumstances here which I'd like to discuss with you. The mother was out and the oldest child, a girl of 13, was babysitting. She fed the baby and put her into her cot. She'd done this before so the mother had no worries about leaving her babysitting and she wasn't gone long. Naturally, they're all devastated. The police have explained to the mother that an autopsy will have to be done and she understands and accepts that.'

He paused. I knew what he was going to ask. I knew it would be the end of my Sunday plans, because I also knew what my answer was going to be. Our spoilt day was nothing compared with what that family would be going through.

'I've been asked if a post-mortem can be done today so they can have her back as soon as possible.'

'Yes, of course. I'll have to make a few arrangements first, but I'll be able to start in an hour or so. We should be finished by mid-afternoon and then they can have her back.'

Cot deaths were always so sad. To see and hold perfectly formed well-cared-for children with no discernible cause of death always seemed an affront to me. The post-mortems were challenging. Not only was there the emotion of opening and examining a perfectly normal, unblemished and beautiful-looking baby, but they were technically difficult too. There are many investigations to be carried out. Besides the routine tests, I had collected blood and tissue for Dr Skinner's lab to look for a QT syndrome. There was the fluid from behind the eye to measure the baby's electrolytes.

At first, I found nothing at all. Everything was normal, as is usual in cot deaths.

'Mr Hubbard, there is nothing to find,' I reported that evening. 'A healthy looking, well-cared-for baby according to everything I've found. Of course, my histology on the tissue slides will take a few days. And there'll be toxicology studies to come, but I'm not expecting to find drugs.'

We both knew that poisoning from cocaine or heroin was quite improbable in a traditional rural family, although you never know for sure.

'Yes, drugs are unlikely,' Graham Hubbard said. 'What about poisons? RoundUp? Anything like that?'

This was a possibility, as most rural families had a range of chemical nasties to hand, such as RoundUp, and any number of other chemical sprays used to control weeds and pests in their crops and pastures.

'It's possible, but I'd have expected to see something in the stomach. I didn't find anything but curdled milk. I've sent the stomach contents off to be analysed, just in case.'

'So what do we reckon for the cause of death?'

I knew he needed something to release the child's body.

'Well, it is a cot death in the absence of anything else.'

'That'll have do for now. So I take it I can release the child?'

'Yes. I have everything I shall need.'

'Good night, then, Doctor, and thanks for your trouble. I know it will be a great comfort to the family to have their wee one back so soon.'

The Cause of Death

* * *

I have done many a heartbreaking autopsy on these infants over the years, but this one sticks in my memory, because there was an answer.

It came from the fluid I had drawn from the eyeball.

When I read it, I gasped. The baby's sodium level was 167 milliequivalents per litre. This level was fatally high. The absolute maximum was 140 milliequivalents and that was for an adult. What on earth could have happened here?

It proved to be an old story.

The baby was not on the breast but was fed formula — powdered milk — which is fine when used as directed. Cow's milk is not a perfect substitute for mother's milk and one problem is that it is full of extra sodium. This is just too much for a child's immature kidneys to handle so the amount given has to be just right.

Apparently, on the night in question, the baby was unsettled and crying. The family had all got into the habit of ignoring the measuring spoons provided and thickening up the formula to make a 'stronger bottle' to help settle her. But too much formula meant too much sodium. Sodium is poisonous, and so she had died. This was a great sadness to us all.

* * *

Another case of sudden death in infancy sticks in my memory, but for very different reasons.

Trouble with the Babysitter

Demis Paul had a colourful life, to put it mildly. He knew the police, and they knew him well, too. Demis was the son of Jan Yorke, who was a Taranaki-based sex-worker trading under the professional name 'Velvet'. She became involved with a married man, and decided that his wife, Nicola Goodwin, was an impediment to their relationship. So she decided to murder her. The police investigation led to Velvet, and she was sentenced to 13 years' imprisonment in 1995.

When I first came across him, Demis had 21 previous convictions for a variety of crimes, including burglary, theft, receiving and possession of an offensive weapon as well as damaging property and endangering life with fire and explosives. He had served part of a 27-month sentence for burglary and drug offences when he applied to be released into home detention. The parole board agreed, so long as someone could be found to take him into their home.

He was accepted into a home where two sisters lived, caring for their three children.

It seemed to be going okay at first. But on the evening of 22 December, the two women had gone to town to join the throng of Christmas shoppers to buy presents for their children, whom they left with Demis.

According to Demis's story, he had bathed the children, fed them their tea and put the 14-month-old girl down on the bed. Hearing a noise a short time afterwards, he went in and to his horror, found the two-and-a-half-year-old boy jumping up and down on his infant cousin's stomach. She was limp and unresponsive. Demis carried out CPR and alerted the neighbours and an ambulance was summoned.

The Cause of Death

The young innocent was dead on arrival in the Emergency Department. It was a sombre team from the CIB that assembled to watch me perform the autopsy at ten the next morning.

There was massive bruising of the abdomen wall, which spoke of a considerable blow. The stomach was full of blood. The bowel was completely torn in two, guillotined between whatever had delivered that fierce blow and the hard, unyielding bone of the spinal column. From the resulting tear, she had bled to death through the ruptured blood vessels.

'What could cause that?' a detective asked.

'A punch or a kick would do it. I've seen it a couple of times in kids who have come off their bikes at speed and landed gut-first on a handlebar. It's a savage force, as it's all concentrated abruptly on a small surface area. And of course, you often see it in high-speed car accidents and aircraft crashes where the seatbelt causes the injury.'

'How about another kid jumping on her stomach? Could that do it?'

I thought a long while about that. I had to concede it was at least a physical possibility. The detectives looked at me sceptically. Like me, many of them were dads with experience of kids at play. They weren't buying it.

There was more to find.

'She had an intussusception of her bowel,' I told them.

'What does that mean?'

'It's not related to the injury. It's not uncommon, but what it means for some kids is they get a minor viral infection and the lymphoid tissue in the bowel wall swells up to combat the virus. The bowel moves all the time, doing a thing called peristalsis — passing food along for digestion. In these infected kids, the bowel drags and tugs on the swollen bowel wall and telescopes the short inflamed tract of gut down into the next bit. It can be silent and cause no effects, but it's often painful. When it is, you get a very distressed, grizzly child.'

The detectives nodded. They could see what I was implying.

Still, in order to move past the explanation we had been given, I had to determine whether a jumping child could have ruptured the bowel. I tried textbooks and journals first. I read that abusive parents often say that their children's bowel perforations were due to falling down stairs. In fact, that's the most common explanation.

Like so much in medical literature, the opinions were divided on the question of whether that was credible. Harvard paediatricians apparently didn't think so. They found that not one of 312 children with perforated bowels had sustained them through accidental trauma. On the other hand, surgeons from Ohio State University thought that half of such cases were caused by minor trauma such as tripping or being fallen on by playmates.

So learned opinion was a stalemate.

I read about two young children wearing adult-sized lap belts in the back seat of a car which had a head-on collision at 30 miles per hour. They both had the identical injury, which was a solitary, small hole punched in their bowel wall. Both holes were in the same place as my child's rupture, although they were much less massive.

The Cause of Death

I wondered whether we could calculate the amount of force that caused those seatbelt injuries and then compare it to the force with which the boy might have subjected her by jumping on her. Would that tell us if the story was credible? It seemed complicated but I decided to try.

I contacted Jim Lewis, the Professor of Physics at Massey University, for help. He certainly thought a meaningful comparison was possible. He produced several pages of mathematical calculations and graphs that gave a result for the force per square centimetre that would be exerted by the seat belts in the reported car crash. That was a start, but how did that compare with the sort of force the young boy could generate by jumping as high as he could then landing with all his weight concentrated in one of his heels?

The police fingerprint expert brought me an imprint of both of his footprints so I could measure the area of his heel. The Wellington paediatric surgeon Kevin Pringle and I examined and weighed him in the outpatients' department in the hospital. We got him bouncing on a bed and found that no matter how much we exhorted him, he could jump no more than 20 centimetres high.

Jim Lewis had built an apparatus in the Massey physics lab that could measure the force from a falling object and the effect of changing the length of time of the impact. That was important. To land with all the force in 1/30th of a second was 30 times more powerful than landing over one second. From this information Jim calculated the absolute maximum force with which the young cousin could have landed on the victim's stomach. It was less than a third of that calculated for the seatbelt accident. On the physical evidence, Demis's story did not stack up.

He heard my evidence in depositions, which was a pre-trial hearing heard before Justices of the Peace. He stuck to his story for the 11 months right up to the time of trial. It was, needless to say, a time of immense distress to the entire family, especially for the young boy's mother, who was racked by guilt. It was a terrible thing that her boy was being blamed for this tragedy, let alone so close to Christmas.

Demis was advised and represented by the very able barrister Duncan Harvey. Six days before the trial, Demis at last confessed to punching the little girl, although he maintained he didn't mean to kill her. It happened exactly as we had speculated. He said she had been fretful and upset that fatal night, crying bitterly from time to time. Her crying was probably due to her painful intussusception of bowel. Demis had lost control and struck her violently with his fist as she lay on the bed wailing.

The jury had no hesitation in finding him guilty of murder.

All he could offer in mitigation was that he had anger problems and didn't know his own strength. Justice Gendall gave that excuse short shrift, and said a crying 14-month-old baby in the care of a person can never be regarded as capable of depriving an ordinary man or woman of their self-control. He sentenced Demis Paul to life imprisonment with a minimum non-parole period of 17 years.

* * *

Justice Gendall also noted that Demis's background was sad, but that this wasn't at all unusual for violent criminal offenders. He is quite correct in this assertion. Demis is a member of a small but sociologically interesting group of murderers, namely those whose parents were also murderers (excluding gang members, where genetic murder is usual and perhaps even compulsory).

In that dismal gallery, Demis joins Dr Colin Bouwer, the former Head of Psychiatry at the University of Otago who murdered his wife by administering diabetic medication to drop her blood sugar to a lethal low. Bouwer's son was separately convicted of a murder in South Africa. I wonder whether such parent–offspring cases are due simply to chance or whether there is some genetic lack of human empathy evident?

Certainly two of the three babysitters in these stories, Heather Ross and Demis Paul, showed a deep and disturbing lack of empathy for the helpless babies entrusted to their care, and the juries thought so too. I am sure that to carry out these deeds must be some form of serious mental illness, but until that is established we have to continue to manage these as crimes.

CHAPTER 11

The Circumstances of Death

Suicide is a dark subject. It was (and is) illegal in many countries, although I'm not sure how one is charged and presumably punished after the act. It's not a subject that we like to talk about and some say the law should forbid even using the word, for fear of copycat suicides. It is illegal to report a suicide as such unless a coroner has expressly so directed. That's what accounts for the range of coded euphemisms that the press use to report it ('there were no suspicious circumstances'; 'police are not seeking anyone else in relation to the incident'). One may not report any of the details or even a suggestion of the method or location of a self-inflicted death.

In this environment, it will always be hard to have a frank and healthy discussion on the topic. To me, it seems a pity, for in New Zealand more than ten people (including one teenager) took their own lives every week during 2016. The Chief Coroner declared this rate to be unacceptably high, and

The Cause of Death

it clearly is. Shaun Robinson of the Mental Health Foundation called for 'courageous conversations' about what is, on the face of it, an epidemic. And none of these discussions touch upon the unresolved debate about assisted euthanasia.

The investigation of suicides is a major part of our day's work. Mostly they are straightforward, but in any death, it is never enough to carry out a post-mortem, find a disease or an injury and call that the cause of death. All the pathological findings have to be looked at in the context of where and how the death occurred. What, that is, were the circumstances? Pathologically speaking, there is little or no difference between a man who has drowned while getting into difficulty swimming, for example, and one who happens to have had a chance heart attack while swimming in the river. It is only the circumstances that will give the answer and tell us the truth.

Many of our cases are deaths from hanging. People often wonder why we bother to carry out autopsies on people who have hanged themselves. It is a good question. Hangings are invariably suicidal, but it is our job to make sure they are not a murder or just a bizarre accident. I always start with the circumstances. Are there any relevant social circumstances such as a divorce or financial troubles? Is there a history of mental illness? What does the scene of death look like? And most importantly, is there a last letter?

Sometimes there is a letter, but it can be difficult to find. Once, early in my career, a policeman and I were investigating what appeared to me to be a suicide, but we were troubled at the fact that, despite a thorough search,

The Circumstances of Death

we couldn't find a letter. The policeman looked around the lounge room, deep in thought. I saw him stop and stare and then walk over to the fireplace, in which paper and kindling was laid ready for a fire to be lit. He reached to the very back and pulled out a crumpled ball of paper. It was the last letter, unfinished.

'How did you know it was there?' I asked in admiration.

'Aw, I just figured, what if you wrote a letter but decided not to leave it? It just seemed the obvious thing to do. Screw it up and chuck it into the fireplace.'

If there is no history and no last letter, then could this be murder? Has the victim been murdered and then hanged to make it look like a suicide? There are clues to find.

We look at the noose mark around the neck — the way in which the pressure of the noose has abraded, indented and dried the skin. It is most pronounced on the side of the neck where the maximum weight is borne, and is the least on exactly the opposite side where the knot holds. And there is often a matching trail of dried saliva out of one side of the mouth. Sometimes there is so much saliva that it had dripped onto the clothing.

Why is this and what does the saliva trail tell?

The rope puts pressure on the pterygopalatine ganglion in the neck, which is a nerve intersection rather like a spaghetti junction on a motorway. One of its major roads leads straight to the salivary glands, so that when the pressure of the rope bears upon this spaghetti junction, a powerful nerve signal travels on upward to stimulate the salivary glands. This means there often is a rush of saliva at death.

The Cause of Death

The presence of this drool proves the person was still alive while he or she was being strangled by the noose, because a body cannot make saliva after death. The victim was therefore not dead at the time of hanging, and no-one is trying to hide a murder by faking a suicide. The saliva trail is always on the opposite side of the mouth to the hanging point because the head always hangs away from that side. It is logical, but it would be a lucky murderer who got everything to look right. Therefore, if those clues are present, QED: it must be a suicidal hanging not a murder. The death is tidy and proven and we can often leave it at that.

Many families and coroners these days ask pathologists to carry out an external examination of hangings and to forgo opening the body. I agree in principle to forgoing an autopsy, provided all the right circumstances are present and everything stacks up.

External autopsies are still controversial, as many forensic pathologists believe that only a full examination will stop us missing critical clues, such as unrecognised pregnancies in young teenagers. I have even heard an Australian forensic pathologist say that he always checks for murder by flaying the skin of the arms to look for hidden bruises left by restraints.

One has to be experienced to understand the pooling of blood or livedo in hangings to ensure the blood is located where it would be expected in a suspended body. It would usually be in the lower legs. But while it is unusual, some hangings are carried out in the sitting position, in which case the blood pools in the buttocks, the legs and the hands.

The Circumstances of Death

I often wonder what motivates a suicidal person to hang themselves in the sitting position. Can they really believe the suffering or pain will be less? Or are they trying in some fumbling way to balance pain and suffering? No-one who hasn't been there can ever really know.

There is also the problem of 'Kirshofrosen', dark blotchy marks on the skin in front of and at the tips of the ears. These are often seen in death from hanging. It is blood pooling after death or during the last, agonal second of life and it looks like bruising. As it is not in a gravity-dependent place like the legs or back or buttocks, the uninitiated might suppose it is from an attack before death. But it is a change uniquely associated with hanging, the natural leaking of blood out into the tissues, and it looks worse after death.

These changes are even harder to accept in accidental hangings, which are rare. Once again, it is the circumstances that tell the story. I had never heard of auto-erotic asphyxia until this type of death was widely publicised by rock star Michael Hutchence's death in a Sydney hotel. From that episode, I learned that some men set up ingenious devices to partially strangle themselves while having an orgasm. The idea is that if the brain is deprived of oxygen at the moment of orgasm, the experience is substantially enhanced. Mostly they use nooses with a 'safety' release mechanism. There are a large number of variations including plastic bags, tape, sacks, anaesthetic chemicals and other methods.

If they are just experimenting, what actually kills them? Well, the room for error is slight. It takes only a second or so to lose consciousness and then there is no time to use the safety procedures. They are caught totally by surprise. One second they experience ecstasy, the very next there is eternal blackness and death.

Is the loss of consciousness through asphyxia always so quick? I have read about condemned prisoners in London dancing the 'Tyburn jig' — struggling for their lives while actually hanging by the neck. Pathologists have learned a great deal about asphyxial deaths from historical executions, and tens of thousands of men, women and even children were publicly hanged at Tyburn. There was no drop from a height as with the more modern judicial executions. The condemned prisoners stood on carts while the crowd sang and danced and even threw horse dung at the victim, chanting: 'Oh, my! Look who's going to die!'

Then the horses would be whipped and the cart would lurch off.

For most, a sudden death was the rule, but the crowds used to howl in disappointment and frustration when the victim did not dance the Tyburn jig. When the victim did buck and kick, relatives would run forward and pull down on their loved one's legs to try to speed up their dying. It sounds horrific, but we no longer believe they were conscious. Most 'dances' were brainstem fits, quite involuntary, running on a dying automatic spasm. Botched hangings did happen, as the quality of ropes was poor and multiple attempts were sometimes made before the hangman's job was done.

The loss of consciousness may be so swift in auto-erotic asphyxias that there is absolutely no possibility of saving oneself from the consequences. The pursuit of the heightened sexual experience is very widely discussed today, so no doubt there is more experimentation than ever. Some say these cases should not be discussed in the public arena for fear they will be copied, but that horse may have already bolted. Hiding this particular activity will not make it go away in today's age of easy information. We must face this openly, and everyone should be aware of the extreme danger and high likelihood of a sudden accidental death in this perilous game.

* * *

I was asked for an opinion in a case in which I was not the pathologist directly involved. One August, as the first lambs were being born to take their chances with a late fall of snow, I was consulted by a senior Queen's Counsel who was representing an insurance company and who was seeking a second pathological opinion.

'How did you get my name?' I asked in surprise. I was, after all, a provincial pathologist in the Manawatu. I was both surprised and pleased to hear that he had been given my name by a defence lawyer who had given me a very hard time under cross-examination in the witness box. Obviously I had done something right.

'What is it you're looking for?'

'My client has a claim they want to contest. It's a case of sudden death and they want an independent pathologist's view. There will, of course, be a professional fee.'

I was seriously pushed for time with my diagnostic commitments — biopsies on living patients and my routine

The Cause of Death

autopsies — and I doubted I'd have time for anything more than to have a quick look at the case and to make a brief comment on its merits.

'How much would the fee be?' I asked.

The lawyer named a figure.

'Yes,' I said straight away. 'I'm happy to help.'

My salary was adequate, but hardly exorbitant.

Fortunately, the case was interesting. It involved a truck driver for a haulage company who had a regular run between small towns. He would unload a delivery, pick up another load for the next destination and then return home. He did the same run, regular as clockwork, for years.

Then, for unknown reasons, he lost his job. As this was a civil case and not a criminal one, there wasn't the same massive power to collect relevant information.

He held a life insurance policy, which was payable if death was accidental. Suicide was specifically excluded, as is usual in these types of contracts. He kept paying his monthly insurance premiums, though it must have been a drain on the family expenses until one day, for no apparent reason, he had a fatal traffic accident.

The striking feature of the accident was that he was driving in the reverse direction on his old trucking route when, on a long, straight part of a state highway in clear daylight, he crossed the centre line and collided head-on with the truck that he had driven for so many years, now being driven by the man who replaced him. He was killed instantly. There were no witnesses to the crash. The truck driver was shaken but unhurt, and maintained that the car definitely veered

The Circumstances of Death

towards him. The insurance company executive who was telling me the story said that the truck driver thought the man in the car was still holding the steering wheel as they collided, but he couldn't be certain.

'That's hardly unexpected,' I said. 'He'd have been in shock. It's a traumatic event.'

'Of course. But what do you think? We don't want to rush in and make a judgement about this.'

I thought about it.

'It seems very odd for an accident,' I mused. 'Did he have any reason to be on that particular stretch of road at that time?'

'No, none at all. It wasn't work-related travel, because he was unemployed at the time.'

'Do we know anything about his mental state? Did he suffer from depression?'

'We don't know. By law, we're not allowed access to his medical information. Our investigator found out he was seeing his GP, but we don't know why.'

'Well, it sounds like suicide to me. What's it exactly you want my opinion on?'

'The local pathologist decided the death was from natural causes. He thought the man was dead before the accident.'

I was interested in that.

'Why?' I asked. 'There must be some scientific basis to that decision. What did his autopsy report show?'

'I'll leave that with you to read. Phone me if you're prepared to act for us.'

* * *

The Cause of Death

The post-mortem report was interesting. It was thorough, well-constructed and clearly came to the conclusion that the death was natural. I knew and respected the pathologist who had written it. His qualifications and experience in pathology were impressive. But I was sure he must be wrong.

The crux of his findings stated there was a large haemorrhage at the base of the brain, situated around the brain stem. There was no associated skull fracture. He believed that this haemorrhage represented an arteriovenous malformation. An arteriovenous malformation is an abnormal growth of arteries and veins supplying blood to the brain and it would have had to be there from birth. When (and if) it ruptures, it can lead to sudden incapacitation or even death. That could have happened at any time of his life, and it so happened it spontaneously ruptured while the man was driving.

I absolutely agreed with all of the findings in the autopsy report, with the exception of the conclusion that an arteriovenous malformation was responsible. I personally was not convinced that the brain haemorrhage came from an arteriovenous malformation. I had seen many similar haemorrhages at the base of the skull sustained in traffic accidents. They are common. They are a result of the force of impact and were never natural diseases causing the accident.

Any rapid, rotational force applied to the head and neck can result in a tear to the vertebrobasilar artery. It is well documented, for example, that a sharp punch to the side of the head can rotate the head on the neck, rupturing the artery. It is particularly common when the victim is drunk.

The Circumstances of Death

In those cases, the victim either does not see the blow coming, or fails to brace his neck muscles in anticipation of the blow, perhaps even both. I have seen just such a case where a nightclub bouncer quite lightly struck a very drunk patron. The degree of force needed is not great in the right circumstances.

The deceased driver was certainly not drunk. His blood alcohol level was zero. But the force of the impact would have been enormous, vastly greater than an unprotected blow from a fist. The effect would be exactly the same.

Could the same argument apply if he happened to have an arteriovenous malformation as a further point of weakness? It is a good question. It could arguably be the same. However in an arteriovenous malformation, I would expect to see a mesh or net of dilated veins and arteries both on the surface of the brain and embedded in the blood clot. I examined the tissue slides taken by the local pathologist. I saw no evidence of any such lesion. The sections were of fresh blood clot only with no blood vessels present.

So could I positively exclude an artery malformation in this case? I thought hard about that. Not absolutely. No-one could honestly do that without a complete examination of the brain. I could only comment on the appearance of the relatively small amount of brain sampled for microscopic examination. But there was certainly none on the slide, of that I was certain, and that was the only evidence remaining.

Once the physical evidence found in a post-mortem or any other pathology investigation has drawn the outlines, you need circumstances to fill in the picture. The evidence always has to be interpreted in the context of the case. What might be true in one context might not be so when considered in another.

Suppose the car had veered off the road and had gradually come to rest totally undamaged on the verge, and he was found dead at the wheel. In that scenario, I could easily accept that this was a natural death arising from a rupture in arteriovenous malformation. But that scenario wasn't the context in this case.

He was on a road for no apparent reason that any of the investigators had been able to find. His car veered suddenly and unexpectedly and collided with the only other vehicle for miles around, which happened to be his old work vehicle belonging to the company from which he had been dismissed. I thought the odds against this constellation of circumstances coming together in one time and place to produce these injuries by a chance natural event must be astronomically huge.

A natural event seemed unlikely. A deliberate act occasioned by a momentary fit of rage seemed far more likely.

In the end, my opinion wasn't accepted. Death was found to be haemorrhage from an arteriovenous malformation, causing him to lose control of the vehicle in which he was driving and collide with an oncoming truck. I was disappointed in a professional sense, although I knew that pathologists become well known to their local coroners who, given a choice, naturally will tend to believe the man they know and trust. Local prejudice then often becomes local wisdom. That is the nature of things.

And as the QC pointed out, the outcome was good for the man's widow. When I thought about her — ageing, alone and with no resources — I could see the bright side of losing the debate. Understanding the human cost of death is not part of our training. That is more narrowly focused on the autopsy findings, but I would have felt terrible if my evidence had caused financial and personal distress to a family already suffering from such a tragic loss.

Remembering there are people at the end of our investigations helps us to keep our humanity.

* * *

WHERE TO GET HELP
Lifeline (open 24/7) 0800 543 354
Depression Helpline (open 24/7) 0800 111 757
Healthline (open 24/7) 0800 611 116
Samaritans (open 24/7) 0800 726 666
Suicide Crisis Helpline (open 24/7) 0508 828 865 (0508 TAUTOKO). This is a service for people who may be thinking about suicide, or those who are concerned about family or friends.
Youthline (open 24/7) 0800 376 633. You can also text 234 for free between 8 a.m. and midnight, or email talk@youthline.co.nz
0800 WHATSUP children's helpline 0800 9428 787, open between 1 p.m. and 10 p.m. on weekdays and from 3 p.m. to 10 p.m. on weekends. Online chat is available from 7 p.m. to 10 p.m. every day at www.whatsup.co.nz

The Cause of Death

Kidsline (open 24/7) 0800 543 754. This service is for children aged 5 to 18. Those who ring between 4 p.m. and 9 p.m. on weekdays will speak to a Kidsline buddy who is a specially trained teenage telephone counsellor.

Your local Rural Support Trust 0800 787 254 (0800 RURAL HELP)

Alcohol Drug Helpline (open 24/7) 0800 787 797. You can also text 8691 for free.

For more information, contact the Mental Health Foundation's free Resource and Information Service on 09 623 4812.

CHAPTER 12

The Smallest Speck of Evidence

'What do you make of this?'

Detective Senior Sergeant Ross Grantham from the CIB handed me a cardboard folder containing a glass slide.

I took the slide and looked at it carefully. Beneath the coverslip was a light smear of stained material.

'What's this all about?' I asked, having learned from long experience that there would be a strange, complex and tragic tale behind the specimen, if it was typical of something the CIB brought me. And sure enough, this was the beginning of a bizarre and complicated case that was to last for years, and one that would take me across the world and back again before being settled in 2015.

'It's something that forensics rubbed onto the slide from a murder suspect's shirt. They think they can see something cellular on the slide, but they're not sure exactly what it is.

The Cause of Death

Can you and your pathologists have a look and see what you think?'

It took me quarter of an hour to go over the slide at high microscopic magnification.

'Well?' said Ross. 'What do you think it is?'

'This looks like brain to me.'

He stared unblinkingly back at me. 'Why?'

'It just looks like brain.'

Ross looked at me sceptically. 'What makes you say that?'

I thought carefully. This wouldn't be easy to explain.

'When a pathologist makes a diagnosis, mostly we recognise what we see instantly. It gets called the "Aunt Minnie" sign.'

'Who the hell's Aunt Minnie?'

'It goes like this. How do you know that an old lady in front of you is your Aunt Minnie? Well, it's usually because you just know. You've seen her hundreds of times before and you know what she looks like and who she is. You don't have to go through the whole scientific rigmarole you'd go through if you didn't recognise her — you know, examine her facial profile, measure her height or count her moles or whatever. Some pathologists call this using the "lizard part" of your brain, the ancient dinosaur bit that runs on automatic without any intelligent thought. Some psychiatrists call the process "gestalt", whatever the hell that is. In the end, I think it means the same thing.'

'It doesn't sound like something we could use in court.'

'Well, no, but you asked me what it was. I've done both things. I've done an Aunt Minnie on it, but I've also cross-checked.'

The Smallest Speck of Evidence

We moved to sit at the multi-headed microscope in the lab. There were three pathologists present, as well as two registrars, and they all had a look at the slide. We all reached the same conclusion.

'We don't have to rely on Aunt Minnie,' I told Ross. 'We can see cells, including a cellular, tubular structure, which is a small blood vessel. That tells us we're looking at deep tissue, deeper than the surface of the skin.'

'What about spit?' asked Ross. 'Or snot from the nose? Could it be from that?'

'No,' I said. 'You'll never find blood vessels in spit, snot, urine or any other body fluids. They have to come from deep tissue. And the cells are all oval with what we call spindle-shaped nuclei. The nuclei are bland in appearance, which means they've had much of their cellular material stripped away. But the background between these cells has a subtle, fibrillary look. It doesn't really fit with anything other than brain tissue. I mean, it's not muscle or thyroid gland or pancreas or spleen or liver. I could go on and on. It's a long list, but I really don't think that this tissue can be anything other than brain.'

The others murmured in agreement.

Ross sat in silence for a very long time, thinking.

Finally he spoke. 'Can you prove it?'

'Prove that it's brain?'

He nodded.

We all looked at each other and one after another we shook our heads.

'No,' I said. 'Not with our resources here. This is the only slide, I suppose?'

The Cause of Death

Ross nodded.

'I thought so. There's not much on it, either. I suppose special stains could be tried, but it would be difficult. Particularly if you are looking for the level of proof you need for a murder case.'

Ross grimaced. I could tell that he really wanted a result on this one. And like most New Zealanders, when they came to hear the terrible facts of the case, I was inclined to agree.

* * *

Mark Lundy was a travelling salesman of kitchen and bathroom ware. He lived in Palmerston North with his wife, Christine, and their seven-year-old daughter, Amber. He was generally regarded as something of a character by his friends, being into amateur dramatics and the Scout movement and having a passion for fine wines.

His business wasn't exactly thriving, so he had conceived a scheme to buy a plot of land in the Hawke's Bay region to convert into a vineyard. He had made an unconditional offer of two million dollars and he had also ordered a considerable number of grapevine saplings for his initial planting. But with little capital of his own and no access to finance, he was counting on attracting investors for his project. They had failed to materialise. Mark and Christine had also taken out insurance policies on one other whereby each stood to receive five hundred thousand dollars in the event of the other's death.

That was the background. It's what happened next that transfixed the nation.

The Smallest Speck of Evidence

Lundy left their Palmerston North home on an overnight business trip to Wellington, where he had some clients to visit. He checked into a motel and at 8.30 p.m. used his cell phone to call an acquaintance, with whom he discussed his business prospects. Then he arranged for the services of a call-girl from one of the local escort agencies. She left his motel unit at about 1 a.m. Over the course of the evening, he had drunk half a bottle of rum.

At 9.30 the next morning, Christine's brother found her body and that of Amber Lundy hacked to death on the floor of their house. They had bought meals from McDonald's at six o'clock the previous evening, and that was the last time they were confirmed to be alive. A window next to the front door had been levered open, suggesting a forced entry.

A friend contacted Mark in Wellington the next morning and he rushed back to Palmerston North. He was intercepted at the outskirts of the city, and taken to the police station. There he was told the horrific news. His clothing, car and contents were seized by the police, as is the usual protocol.

The autopsies on the brutalised bodies of mother and daughter were performed by my colleague James Pang, an experienced pathologist in Palmerston North. He was able to say that the weapon was most probably an axe, and he found multiple flakes of blue and orange paint deeply embedded in the wounds as well as in fragments of skull bone lodged in Christine's head. These were assumed to have come from the murder weapon.

He also found that the stomachs of both Christine and Amber contained apparently undigested food, which he believed was recognisable as fish and chips. That was thought to be consistent with the food ordered from McDonald's. There was apparently no food in the duodenum of either victim. Since the process of gastric emptying hadn't begun, James concluded that death had occurred about one hour after eating.

Forensic clues started to paint an interesting picture. Blood was found on the outside of the latch of the open window, and this proved to be Christine's. The supposed break-in appeared to have been staged. There was less petrol in Mark Lundy's car than there should have been, if it had been driven only on the detailed itinerary he had voluntarily compiled for the police, and the indications were that the car had travelled 400 kilometres further than Lundy claimed. He tried to explain the discrepancy away, saying that there had been talk of thefts of petrol from cars around the area he'd stayed in the Lower Hutt motel. If there was any shortfall in petrol, he told the investigating officers, then that would have to be the explanation.

Mark Lundy's tools were all painted in a distinctive orange and blue. There was a full set of tools in his garden shed, but no axe. Lundy maintained that he didn't own an axe — an assertion contradicted by several of his acquaintances.

Nor was his subsequent behaviour that which you might expect of the bereaved husband and father of the victims of a brutal murder. Lundy claimed he went every night to his girls' graveside to have a drink with them, but he couldn't prove he had done so. On the contrary, he spent a good deal of time socialising, drinking, buying expensive motorbikes and, more bizarrely, even continued his enjoyment of call-girl services.

When I learned this last detail, I shook my head in disbelief. I had seen plenty of grieving relatives over the years, and had known some of them to react in bizarre ways. I had only to remember the widower in my weird exhumation case. I knew that it didn't prove Mark Lundy had done it, although it certainly revealed that he had an unusual and dark side. But his behaviour seemed extreme, by any standard.

Others were reaching the same conclusions. Lundy's physical collapse at Christine and Amber's funeral, which was shown almost nightly on television for several days, struck many people as melodramatic and unconvincing. A psychologist stated in the media that he was firmly of the opinion that the display of grief was contrived.

A witness came forward saying she had seen a large man with an unusual gait wearing a blond wig running along the road away from the Lundy house just after 7 p.m. on the night of the murders. He had a horror-struck look on his face. It turned out that the witness was a psychic.

The case was avidly followed and discussed in workplaces all around the country, and the Palmerston North mortuary was no exception.

'Psychologists and psychics! What next?' I laughed to my colleagues. 'Why, with all that help, do the police even need a pathologist?'

The answer was yes, they certainly did. The police needed to know exactly what was on Mark Lundy's shirt.

The Cause of Death

* * *

We asked why the slide was only being presented now. After all, the murders had been committed a couple of months previously, on 29 August 2000. We were told the ESR forensics lab had a punishing workload and no immediate priority was given to Lundy's clothes. The shirt had been kept for examination, and when they got around to it 59 days after the crime, they found three spots of blood. One was on the upper-front of the left-hand side of the shirt and a second on the upper-left sleeve. Both tested positive for Christine's DNA. The third on the lower-right side of the shirt contained Amber's DNA. The forensic scientist moistened up the biggest stain with saline and then dabbed it onto the glass slide.

This was the famous 'dab' slide that we were examining and that we all thought was brain tissue.

How could we reach the level of scientific certainty necessary to stand up in court? Could we get more tissue off the shirt to make a more definite identification? Talking it over, we thought it might be possible if the ESR scientist had not rubbed all the material off, but it was beyond our laboratory expertise to do so. We thought an international expert was needed.

The best evidence would be immunological stains to prove it was brain. Our minds turned to Rod Miller, a pathologist in Texas who had been a very impressive guest lecturer at our scientific conference in Palmerston North in 2000, a short while before the murders. Rod is a brilliant scientist and an

The Smallest Speck of Evidence

expert in using immunohistochemistry on tissue samples. We recalled how he told us he had been able to lift cells off a slide and get conclusive immunohistochemistry stains to work. Could he do that with the dab slide? We suggested to Ross that he contact Rod Miller.

That was really all I could do. It was beyond any of our capabilities to do specialist work on the shirt. I did not expect to be involved professionally with the Lundy case again. But like everyone else, I was following it with bated breath.

* * *

Midway through the trial, Ben Vanderkolk, who was prosecuting, telephoned me.

'I need your advice on a development in the Lundy case.'

The trial of Mark Lundy had commenced in Palmerston North in 2002 and was being followed by the nation even more avidly than *Shortland Street*. Like everyone else, most of my information was from the news, fed out in dribs and drabs as the case meandered and the court worked its way through a host of witnesses. I heard that Rod Miller, the international expert from Texas, had come up with the goods. He had positively identified brain tissue from two of the spots on Mark Lundy's shirt. To me it sounded like a compelling piece of evidence for the prosecution.

'As you may have heard,' Ben said, 'Christine Lundy's brain tissue and DNA has been found on Mark Lundy's shirt. This is damning evidence and now the defence are doing pretty much what I would expect.'

'Alleging contamination?' I correctly guessed.

According to Ben, the defence raised two possible methods of contamination. The first was that a piece of brain tissue accidentally got onto the camera lens in the mortuary, was not noticed and the lens was not cleaned. Then, when the photographer was taking photographs of the shirt 18 hours later, the defence suggested that the two small specks of brain fell from the lens and became embedded in the fibres of the shirt.

I was puzzled. 'How would brain tissue get on a lens in the mortuary? The photographers don't handle tissue.'

'Oh, they're saying that when the pathologist pulls his rubber gloves off at the end of the autopsy it's possible that pieces of brain could be catapulted into the air, particularly if the gloves are stretched and flicked about like an elastic band.'

'But that's ridiculous surely? I've never seen any pathologist do that. And anyway you can't do that with those gloves. They are tight-fitting surgical rubber gloves and you have to peel them off inside-out from the cuff down to the fingers. That means any blood and tissue is trapped on the inside, so you can't flick tissue off a glove even if you tried.'

Still, I had to concede it was a novel and interesting defence, and for a conviction to be safe, all possibilities had to be considered. But there was more to come.

Ben went on. 'As I said they have raised a second possibility. Want to take a guess what that is?'

'I've no idea. What else is there? Has the defence actually accepted that it is brain tissue?'

'Yes we believe so, although they haven't said so in as many words. They've had the photographs examined by Beth Synek in Auckland and the slides by Peter Vanezis, a Professor of Forensic Pathology in Glasgow, who agrees it's brain. They haven't yet contested that there's brain tissue present. So we reckon they must have accepted it.'

'Then I don't know. So?'

'They have asked the police whether they deliberately put the brain there on the shirt the next day or at some later point.'

'Mmm,' I pondered. 'That's a pretty serious allegation. Have they got any evidence to back this up?'

'No,' said Ben. 'They're just fishing. It's a pretty weak defence, but I guess they know they're in a difficult position.'

'And what has all this got to do with me?'

'Can you comment on how likely the defence scenario of deliberate contamination is? I mean, from looking at Rod Miller's material and the original dab slide.'

I agreed to have a look at Rod's results and give my opinion. This was now quite a different question from where I had left the case. All those months ago, the issue was how to prove the tissue on the shirt was brain. The new question posed was whether the brain tissue Rod Miller had lifted from the shirt could have been placed there as late as 18 hours after death.

* * *

'The Court calls Dr Temple-Camp!' The crier's booming voice echoed through the building. I went forward and stood in the witness box. The crier peered searchingly into my eyes as usual to make sure I understood the gravity of the occasion, administered the oath, and then took the Bible from me.

'Good morning, Doctor,' said the judge. He had a genial and kindly face. 'Thank you for joining us,' he said courteously, ignoring the fact that I was there under a subpoena. 'I believe the learned counsel here today may wish to ask you a few questions. I would be obliged if you could speak clearly and slowly as our court stenographers do have to keep a complete record. You will appreciate that they do not necessarily have an extensive command of the medical lexicon. But I do feel sure that we will manage between us.' He smiled pleasantly.

Ben Vanderkolk rose and led me through my evidence quickly, efficiently and with precision. I had to admire his performance. He made every effort to put me at my ease so that I could present what I had to say to both the jury and the judge. I could see that he had the full attention of the court. It went well, very well. No-one in the jury was asleep; all eyes were intent on Ben.

In answer to his meticulously constructed set of questions, I described how I had re-studied the original dab slide, which was exactly as I remembered it, and then turned to the slide preparation Rod Miller had made. Rod's slide was breathtaking and quite conclusive. There was plenty of material present and it was instantly recognisable as glial tissue from the brain, complete with fine neural processes running in a complex net through the background tissue.

The Smallest Speck of Evidence

The brain tissue was well-preserved and utterly compelling, trumping the original dab slide totally.

I did not believe the 18-hour planting scenario was possible.

'Why?' Ben asked.

'The critical answer lies in the remarkable preservation of the tissue in Professor Miller's preparation,' I replied, and went on to explain that pathologists use a technique called 'fixation' to preserve human tissue. As soon as any tissue is removed from the body it is effectively dead and begins to rot — the same process that happens when a person dies and the body decomposes. We stop this decay by fixing the tissue, usually with a preservative chemical named formalin. But other chemicals can be used as well, even common table salt.

'I presume the tissue on the shirt wasn't preserved by chemical means,' Ben said. 'Do you mind telling the court how it was preserved?'

'By drying.'

Drying out tissue works fine as a preservative, too. We use it every day in hospitals for tissue needle biopsies — where a kind of core sample of tissue is taken by inserting a hollow needle into a suspect area. We — not just pathologists — also use drying to make and preserve dried fruit and meat. Mummies in the desert were fixed by desiccating them in the dry air.

'In the case of the tissue on the shirt,' I said, 'the brain was sort of mummified onto the shirt. This was a process not unlike that which happens when an insect splatters over a car windscreen. The insect's tissue gets smeared thinly, the wind dries it and it becomes preserved there. It'll still be there months later if it isn't scrubbed off and it will stay surprisingly recognisable.'

'So if drying was the method of preservation, how quickly did that have to happen?' Ben asked.

'I could see the brain architecture very clearly,' I replied. 'It wasn't quite up to textbook standards, but it was pretty close. I suspected the brain tissue had to have been fixed very quickly indeed.'

'Do you have any way of knowing how quickly? And what in your opinion, is the significance of your tests for the tissue found on the accused's shirt?' Ben asked.

'The brain tissue must have been smeared on the shirt pretty much at the time of death,' I replied firmly. 'Certainly within 30 minutes of it.'

'What do you say to the suggestion that the tissue found its way onto the shirt 18 hours after the time of death?'

'It's not credible,' I said. 'The piece of brain we were looking at was far too small to have sat around for 18 hours.'

I had considered, but was not called upon to comment in the trial, whether it might be possible to keep a large chunk of brain and plant a small sample on the shirt 18 hours later to produce the kind of results that we saw under examination. But it's not quite that easy. A large chunk of brain won't dry out as rapidly, but it will decay before it has dried enough to be preserved. Brain tissue decays very rapidly. Even the ancient Egyptians scooped out the brain through the nose as a first step before they mummified a body.

The Smallest Speck of Evidence

A small insect splattering over a windscreen will smear thinly and dry quickly. But if it is something larger — like, say, a small bird — it won't smear or stick and will end up rotting. It is the same with pressing dried flowers in a book. It works well with small delicate flowers, but a big, full-bloomed rose will not dry in the same way. It can't dry out fast enough and will rot into mushy compost.

The tissue on the shirt was a very lucky break for the prosecution. The smear had to be small enough to spread, to dry and to be preserved and also to escape detection by the murderer. A larger smear would have attracted attention and the murderer would have got rid of the shirt. As in the story of *Goldilocks and the Three Bears*, everything had to be just right.

I had thought about how the tissue came to be there in the first place, why there were only two tiny fragments and how it came to be smeared to just the correct degree. I wasn't asked this in court, but a journalist did put it to me subsequently.

After all, given how widely blood and brains were splattered around both the victims, surely there should have been abundant, recognisable blood and brain on the shirt?

I explained to the journalist that the murderer would have taken care to wear protective overalls, anticipating that blood, at the very least, might get onto their clothing. That would explain why the shirt was essentially clean. But if a right-handed murderer were wearing a pair of one-piece denim overalls of the type worn by council rubbish collectors or hospital porters, the first thing they would do, after undoing the fastenings from the top to the bottom, is put their right thumb under the left lapel and peel the sleeve over the shoulder and along the left arm.

If there were a small fragment of brain tissue on the right thumb, one would inevitably have to touch it to the shirt over the left breast and then on the left shoulder as the overalls were pulled off. The touch would be light and glancing rather than a firm and vigorous rub.

What's more, the right thumb is precisely the place I would predict a right-handed axe-murderer to pick up a piece of brain. And taking off his overalls is precisely the way in which he would spread the tissue thinly enough to ensure quick drying and long-term preservation.

That is what I believe happened that night.

* * *

'Thank you, Doctor,' Ben said. 'Those are all the questions I have. Would you mind answering a few questions for my learned friend?' He turned and held his hand out in a gesture of introduction to the defence counsel, Mike Behrens.

Mike Behrens was a tall, dark and lugubrious man with penetrating eyes, pretty much a legend amongst defence counsel. He was an intellectual man of the people, well known for his passionate defence of the disadvantaged, the desperate and the indigent. Respected for his biting cross-examination, he was a man of undisputed honour, honesty and integrity, and he later took those same qualities to the bench.

The Smallest Speck of Evidence

I looked at him and he looked back at me. Our eyes locked. I could see immense intelligence behind the glare. I girded myself mentally for the challenge. I think I was actually looking forward to being cross-examined.

It started easily enough: straightforward questions, easily answered, nothing contentious. And then a question arose which really had me stumped.

'This evidence you are now giving that limits the timing of the deposit of the material on the shirt did not appear in your original brief, did it, Doctor? Surely you would have said so if you believed it at the time. It's a "killer blow", isn't it?'

What was the 'original brief' to which he was referring? I had never given written evidence when I had first examined the dab slide, nearly 14 months beforehand. I realised that the defence were comparing a first draft of the affidavit I had prepared at Ben's request with the final draft written a day later, after I had fully investigated the issue. It is an occupational hazard in homicide investigations that any preliminary comments, rough notes or drafts will be sifted through and minutely compared by astute defence lawyers. They will search for any changes in wording and these will be used to raise the spectre of reasonable doubt. A wise pathologist keeps his thought to himself until the evidence is ready in its final form.

But despite being momentarily discomfited by this question, I felt I had got my evidence across. There were two, vital questions in relation to the stain on the shirt. Rod Miller had answered the first: it was brain tissue. The second was addressed to me: how much time could elapse between the death of the victim and the deposit of the tissue on the shirt?

I explained that I had anticipated the court's need to know exactly how long would it take before brain tissue becomes unrecognisable. I didn't know and the textbooks didn't say. So I did an experiment to find out.

'The fragment of brain on the shirt was less than half a millimetre in size,' I told the jury, 'so I tested how long you can leave half-millimetre pieces of rat brain out in the open before one can no longer smear it thinly enough to remain recognisable.'

The answer, I told them, was surprising. It would take a maximum of 30 minutes. Any longer than that and either the tissue would not spread thinly, or it would spread but be unrecognisable as brain tissue.

I believed that I had answered the question.

The jury understood it all right. The brain matter was on the shirt and that was indeed a killer blow, just as Mike Behrens had described it. Mark Lundy was found guilty and sentenced to 17 years. He appealed, but had his conviction confirmed and had an additional two years added to his sentence by the Court of Appeal, who seemed to think the trial judge had been too lenient.

* * *

For many who had followed the case so closely, that wasn't the end of the matter. Everyone knew the arguments for the prosecution backwards, complete with its flaws. The matter that most exercised armchair analysts was the tight timing of Mark Lundy's dash from Lower Hutt to Palmerston North, which had to be squeezed between phone calls he definitely made in Lower Hutt and the sighting made by the psychic of a panicked man in a wig running from the scene a little later in the evening.

I entered the mortuary one day and overheard Bruce snap at another of our mortuary assistants, Paddy: 'He never could! There's no way you can drive from Wellington to Palmerston North and back in that time and do a murder as well! I mean, it stands to reason. I drive that road all the time and I tell you there's no way he could've driven fast enough in that traffic. I just wish you'd bloody listen. I've already told you twice.'

'Aye, but you only drive at 80 kilometres an hour!' countered Paddy. 'I could do it easy in my car.'

'And I'm not saying he didn't do it,' Bruce seethed. 'The murder, I mean. He might have. Probably did. I'm just saying he couldn't have driven from Wellington to Palmy at seven o'clock at night, done the murders and got back so fast. Why didn't he do it later, after midnight?'

Paddy shook his head vigorously in denial and opened his mouth to argue back.

I decided to put a stop to this one before the thunder and lightning brewed up.

'That's the trouble with both opinions and arseholes, isn't it, gentlemen?' I said.

'What would that be, Doc?' Bruce looked at me suspiciously.

'Well, everybody has one, don't they? Now let's get on with the work.'

I heard this particular argument again and again over the years. At every dinner party, at every get-together, somebody would surely bring up this topic. University students in the lower North Island even made a joke of it, inaugurating a pub crawl between Wellington and Palmerston North that they named the 'Lundy 500', after a long-standing, analogous event in the South Island named the 'Undy 500'.

It was one of those celebrity cases, and it looked like it would take a very long time before it went away. Together with Rod Miller and others, I published a learned article on our methodology and findings in the Lundy case in the *Journal of Forensic Pathology*. That, I thought, would be that.

CHAPTER 13

Accidents, Accidents, Accidents

I heard the sound of singing as I headed down the steps towards the basement mortuary.

It was beautiful and haunting.

I opened the door and went in.

Farewell ye dungeons dark and strong
　The wretch's destinie!
MacPherson's time will not be long
　On yonder gallows-tree

It was Paddy singing 'MacPherson's Farewell' by Robbie Burns. Paddy was a middle-aged Irishman, content to be an assistant in the mortuary, a quiet worker whom we all liked very much. Paddy was just one of the extraordinarily diverse range of personalities who seemed to gravitate to this type of work. There were comedians and conversationalists and there was even the occasional conspiracy theorist. They came and went, flowing and ebbing around the core of a couple of old time stalwarts. For the job often seemed to attract the itinerant sort of characters who preferred the unpredictable nature of the work to the boring routine of a conventional job. In some ways we are like plumbers, but instead of sewerage, we are there to manage the effluent of death. We sanitise death for society. It's a job quite unlike any other.

All the same, Paddy was the only mortuary singer I ever came across. Today, as he mopped the floor, pushing the water this way and that, he was in full voice:

Sae rantingly, sae wantonly
Sae dauntingly gaed he:
    He play'd a spring and danced it around
    Below the gallows-tree.

'Good morning, Paddy. What have you got for us today? Sounds like a hanging?'

The unexpected was always waiting for our attention. Too often they were the victims of accidents where tragedy not only tore apart bodies, but people's lives as well. Sometimes, though, even accidents could appear to be tranquil, such as this one, which solved the mystery of the disappearance of Arjun Krishnan.

Arjun Krishnan was a happy, 17-year-old school student when he disappeared from his home in Palmerston North,

Accidents, Accidents, Accidents

never to be seen alive again, on 23 January 1985. He had called his mother at 11 that morning to say that he'd be at soccer practice from six to seven o'clock that evening and would stop off at the Lido swimming pool on his way home. But he didn't come home, and when she enquired, his mother learned he hadn't made it to his soccer practice either. His disappearance was completely out of character. An extensive search drew a blank.

Later, in March, a bicycle matching Arjun's was found in the foothills of the Tararua Ranges, not far from Palmerston North. It was lying beneath some ponga tree fronds. Its identification number was misread and the match was not made. The trail then ran cold for the next six years.

A reconstruction of these events was aired on *Crimewatch* in 1991, in which a woman recognised Arjun's distinctive wristwatch as the weather-damaged one found in the bush by her husband while out possum hunting years before.

The police investigation focused once more on the Tararua Ranges. A search team travelled up the Hall Block Road. It is a narrow, unsealed road winding up spectacular, densely forested mountainside. The forest is studded with heavy fans of ponga trees. The moisture-laden westerlies catch on these ranges and it is often clagged in cloud and appears misty, eerie and very much as it might have looked for the last thousand years. When the summit is clear, the giant turbines from the Tararua Wind Farm can be seen scattered along the ridges, scything the air. From the top, you can look back over the Tararua farmland or forward over the entire Manawatu.

It is a beautiful place.

The Cause of Death

And high up here, lying on a heavily forested ridge, the search team found a skeleton.

Here it seemed was Arjun, found at last.

My colleague Bruce Lockett meticulously examined the scene and the position of the skeleton. It was fully clothed and lying on its back, in all respects consistent with a peaceful death, although the skull was found a couple of metres down the slope. Arjun was gently lifted up — nothing was missed, rather like an archaeological dig — and he was carried back to the mortuary. He wasn't home yet, but he was in our care and on his way.

Human bones and pathology have a long association, although during our training, virtually no attention was paid to this important field. We were so overwhelmed with cutting up and examining the bodies of the recently dead that scant attention was paid to the bones of those who had been at rest rather longer. Archaeologists knew far more about how to investigate bones than we did. Nevertheless, we had a job to do, and we had to manage and learn on the job with the help of a few rather basic textbooks.

The clothing was carefully removed for forensic examination and each bone was examined, cleaned and laid out in its anatomically correct position on the table. The skull had a patina of clinging green rootlets and dark earth. Once clean, it was a finely boned, ivory orb. There were no injuries to be seen.

The result was an almost complete skeleton. All that was missing was the third cervical vertebra from the neck.

'Where do you reckon it's got to?' I asked Bruce Lockett.

Accidents, Accidents, Accidents

'No idea. Animals, maybe?' Bruce shook his head. Animal damage from scavengers, rodents and birds was a frequent cause of post-mortem injuries to bodies.

'Could it be a hanging?' I asked. 'I recall reading of a case where after some months the rope eventually cut through the spinal column. The skull was decapitated, and a couple of cervical vertebrae were lost in that one, too.'

We considered it, but the absence of any suitable tree in the vicinity eliminated the possibility. In the end, we thought time and the weather and the runoff of rain rushing down the slope was the explanation for the loss.

The calculation of height is not as straightforward as simply measuring the skeleton. The soft tissue and cartilage has gone, for a start. These days, forensic pathologists measure all of the bones, which they do in a standard way, and consulting a variety of tables, can produce a composite result. We had no access to that degree of sophistication in the early 1990s, although we could use single bones, such as a forearm, to get a rough result. The femur was the most reliable, and based on this evidence, we were able to estimate a height of about 180 centimetres.

The next task was to determine the gender. This can be difficult, although the experts can get it right nearly 100 per cent of the time if they have the whole skeleton. There are narrow, sciatic notches in the pelvis and differences in the femurs, but the skull is the most useful. In a male, the muscle attachments are easier to see and to feel, the mastoid bone behind the ear is bigger and the palate is more U-shaped. We were pretty confident the features we were looking at were male.

The Cause of Death

The age of the person is what everyone asks next. Human bones have growth plates at their ends, which is how we grow taller when young. As we finish growing, these plates fuse solid and we cease to get taller. Fortunately for forensic pathology, this happens at separate but predictable times in different bones. X-rays showed all the plates were fully or nearly fully fused, except for those in the ulna bones at the wrists and the iliac crests on the outer pelvic rim. This gave an age range of 17 to 19, which was close enough.

'What's his racial group? Pakeha or Indian?' the police asked.

No matter how much information a pathologist can provide, the police always seem to have yet one more question, and then one more, until they are sure the well is really dry.

'No idea. The differences are trivial as there has always been a lot of mixing, so it's pretty well impossible to tell. Experts may have opinions but they are often proved to be wrong.'

'And how long has he been dead?'

This was another impossible question to ponder.

'Probably years, but not decades, from looking at the state of the clothing as much as anything else. Sometimes soft tissue decay can happen quickly, so it could be as little as months.'

As pathologists, our primary interest was the cause of death. There were no fractures and no clue as to the cause that we could find. Could this have been an unexpected medical event — an unexpected heart arrhythmia, perhaps? There was no way of knowing at this late stage. Could some

Accidents, Accidents, Accidents

distant hunter firing at a deer accidentally hit and kill a man unknowingly by the merest mischance? But no bullet was found in the surrounding soil. Could it have passed through and left no clue? Was it some other bizarre type of accident that was inconceivable to anyone who wasn't present at the time of death? Pathologists so often find themselves in this difficult space.

We just didn't know, but Arjun could now at last go home to his family.

The coroner ruled that death was due to medical misadventure or an accident.

When I first met Arjun's mother, Ganga, she surprised me by hugging me.

'I wanted him just to come walking home one day,' she told me. 'But at least it's better to have found him and to have him back, even if we'll never know exactly what happened.'

* * *

Accidents cause much of a pathologist's work and sometimes the accidents are so strange that there is no standard way to deal with the investigations. One just has to use common sense and work it out along the way. Some are never solved, of course, such as the mysterious death of Rutger Hale, who was killed by a small, unidentified flying object that came through his car windscreen near Wanaka in 2013. And some accidents have unexpected endings.

The finding of Arjun was a fine thing we could do for his family, but our job was made so much easier by having his whole skeleton on which to identify him. Often we had much less, as little as a single bone, in some cases. One of my most embarrassing cases involved just such a situation.

'Doctor, we have a shoe with something in it for you,' said Patrick, who was on duty one Monday morning.

I'd never had a shoe for autopsy before. One of our pathologists had once been given a left shoe containing part of a foot, which had been found on Foxton Beach. He had been able to get a DNA sample from the tissue and make a positive identification of a missing fisherman. I'd learned in this job that there was always a first time for anything, and I was keen to emulate my colleague's success and find an elegant solution to the case.

'It came from the beach yesterday afternoon,' Patrick said. 'A woman was walking her dogs. Dalmatians, apparently. They found a shoe and kept worrying at it, wouldn't leave it alone, even when she called them. She wondered if there was a foot inside because her dogs wouldn't leave it, so she called the cops on her mobile. They bagged it and sent it through to us. Couldn't be arsed looking for themselves, I reckon. "Just send it to the mortuary. Let them figure it out."'

I occasionally got odd detritus from the beach. There are ossuaries of bones scattered on the sand, and beach walkers and others would hand in suspicious examples to the police. Mainly they came from seals, but also occasionally sheep, cattle, dogs and birds. I had never yet had a human one.

One of my favourite stories, and one that I often used to rib the police with, came from a beach finding. A constable, new to the force, earnestly presented me with the bones of

Accidents, Accidents, Accidents

a seagull wing, which had been crammed by some random mischance of tide or oceans, into a rubber glove. Or maybe it had been deliberately stuffed in there by some kids?

'D'you reckon it's human?' he asked me solemnly.

'Are you serious?' Surely he could see it was a bird?

Were the police trying to wind me up, I wondered? I was suddenly suspicious. I thought that it might not be beyond some of the characters in the CIB to try a practical joke on me.

'I am serious, Doctor,' the young constable said. 'Do you think they're human?' He seemed genuine. I wondered if he was also being set up for a fall. There were feathers still attached, for God's sake.

I decided to wind him up.

'Yes, it's significant. Could be important. Better open a file just in case. You just never know. And you'd better be the officer in charge of the body since you've got custody.'

He left carrying the glove, bones and feathers locked into a small valise. It looked as if this might be his first case.

I had an irritable call about an hour later from a CIB officer. 'Doctor, why are you doing this? What's this nonsense? I've got a very excited policeman in here with a glove full of feathers wanting to start a homicide investigation. Are you serious?'

So it wasn't a joke, after all, but an official inquiry. It was a bit embarrassing. Sheepishly, I had to confess I was just winding him up. I was lucky I wasn't charged with wasting police time.

The shoe was sitting, suspicious and solitary, on the bench.

I approached it thoughtfully.

A trainer shoe, multi-coloured, very pretty: lilac, green, orange. Too pretty to be a serious trainer. More like a fashion item.

The tongue was swollen and salt-stiffened, an ugly protrusion jutting out at me. The whole was encrusted with sand. There was a smell — of seaweed, and … prawns, perhaps?

I sniffed carefully, as if it were a glass of fine wine.

No, not prawns. It reminded me a bit of a Morton Bay bug aroma. Was that a hint of ammonia?

I sniffed again. No.

Could it be human? I wasn't sure.

There was a bone, one bone in the shoe. It was a bit odd, but looked like a metatarsal bone. It looked human, and that it might be from the third toe.

Patrick was subdued now. 'What do you reckon? What does it mean?'

'Well, obviously there must have once been a body attached to the foot from which this bone has come. But there's only one bone left now. It'll be enough, though. We might be able to find who this is from the DNA.'

'What do you need now?' Pat was as usual alert, getting everything precisely right.

'I need the camera to photograph the shoe and bone. I must measure the bone and have it X-rayed. And then I must take a small piece to keep for DNA testing.'

'Okay. Will do.' Pat was off like a dynamo, bringing me a camera, preparing a tray for a tissue sample and getting on the phone to order an X-ray.

Accidents, Accidents, Accidents

I was not entirely sure about the bone, so I decided to take it up to the vet school at Massey University in the morning to see what they thought.

I took photographs of the shoe home that night. I had an idea to make me shine in this investigation.

* * *

'Victoria,' I asked my daughter after tea. 'Can you help me with this shoe?' I handed over the photograph.

She studied it for a while, frowning. 'Where has this come from?'

'It was found on the beach. What I need to know is, what is it? And who might wear it?'

Victoria was a fashion junkie. She followed everything and there was nothing she didn't know about current clothes and shoes and trends.

'That's easy. It's a Sketchers shoe. From about three years ago. I think they were a series called "Pretty Please" or something like that.'

'Who would wear something like that?'

'Not me,' Victoria said firmly. 'Definitely not my style. In fact, none of my friends would wear this style of shoe.'

'So they're quite cheap, are they?'

'Oh no! Daddy, you don't get any shoes cheaply. They're not cheap. I mean, can you guess what this pair of shoes costs?' Victoria tapped the photograph.

'I don't know.' I thought back to the last pair I had bought for myself. 'I suppose about forty dollars?'

Victoria laughed and clapped her hands in glee. 'Nooo! You're absolutely crazy! You really have no idea, do you? Not in this century! Forty dollars? Never! One hundred and twenty dollars a pair at least. That's what you'd pay.'

'Wow! Really? So much just for trainers?'

'Oh yes, but they're more than trainers. They're a fashion statement and they're definitely not cheap. But this particular style?' Victoria frowned as she thought. 'Only 15- to 16-year-old girls would wear these. Maybe they'd have body piercings. Or tattoos. And smoke cigarettes. Out with the boys in their hot cars. That sort of group.'

'Three years ago?' I questioned. 'You're sure?'

'Sure. It was about then. You don't really see that style around much any more.'

Where do all these expensive shoes go when they're not in fashion anymore? One hundred and twenty dollars worn for one year, then gone. Where? How can that be? My shoes were always, easily, still good after ten years. I shook my head sadly. Like most men, I was out of touch for sure.

So much for the philosophical issues. The more gratifying consideration was that Victoria had delivered. I had some quality information for the enquiry.

* * *

'The deceased is female, 15 to 16 years of age, foot size six, probably 165 centimetres tall. Bit of a party girl, decile four to five socio-economically. Possibly with body piercings and maybe a tattoo. Disappeared three years ago.'

Accidents, Accidents, Accidents

I had phoned the constable who had brought in the shoe.

I added that she wasn't local. I knew that because no-one answering that description had disappeared from these parts three years ago. I had visions of a missing teenager lost in a terrible North Island river, car or boating accident and now, at last, I would be the one to find her.

The police officer sounded very sceptical. Who could blame him, with only a shoe and one bone to go on?

Anyway the DNA might yet give the answer. We would just have to wait.

Later that day, I watched the Massey veterinary pathologist easily and positively identify a seal bone. My heart sank with embarrassment.

Definitely not an accident then.

'Idiot!' I told myself. 'I should have checked with the vets first.' But I have to say it did look surprisingly human, even in hindsight. I also made a promise to myself that I would stop playing detective and stick to pathology. Honours between the police and me were now even: the bird's wing to me, the seal bone to them. One-all.

* * *

'Who wants to talk to me?' I asked, mildly taken aback.

'The Hinch programme,' Steve Cordner repeated. 'You know, from Australia?

'I know it,' I confirmed. 'I'm just surprised they want to talk to me.'

The Cause of Death

It was 1992. Professor Steve Cordner was from the Victorian Institute of Forensic Medicine, and he had phoned with the news that journalists for Derryn Hinch's Australian current affairs show wanted to interview me. It was a rarity for the media to want to talk to a pathologist. They generally did not know what we did or, in many cases, even that we existed. Would Hinch himself come to Palmerston North? It seemed improbable. What could be that important?

In the event, it was New Zealand TV journalist Mark Sainsbury who arrived with a cameraman. I supposed he was Hinch's local 'ring-in', though there are few in Auckland who would regard the Manawatu as local. The lab staff were agog and hanging around the corridors as close as they dared. They, of course, recognised Mark with his distinctive, flamboyant moustache as he came through our door. There was a sense of occasion. Palmerston North didn't see many celebrities, let alone the mortuary. We did not attract celebrities very often.

'You might remember three autopsies you did in a traffic accident in April of 1990? It involved a car in a head-on collision with a truck.'

'I think so. Go on.'

Mark consulted his notes briefly.

'Michael Mezzatesta and his wife, Diane, came here on holiday from Melbourne with a friend. So here's the thing.' Mark leaned closer. 'When Michael died, all his money, apparently quite a significant amount, was to go to his wife, Diane, who was also in the car. If she then died, it was to go to her family. If both Michael and Diane died simultaneously, it was to go to Michael's brother.'

Mark paused and pulled a face.

'So basically, depending on the precise timing of each of their deaths, the money either goes entirely to Diane's family or, alternatively, it all goes to Michael's brother and his family. Can we do an interview?'

It turned out to be a fairly complicated case, but I thought I had it. I agreed to give it a go. I smoothed my hair and prepared myself.

Mark shook his head. The interview couldn't be in my office. It was too small, too pedestrian, too boring. There was no library of books to show how clever we were. Lawyers, now — they always look awesome with their walls and walls of gorgeous leather-bound books.

* * *

The interview couldn't be in the mortuary either. Sure, it was the logical place to interview a pathologist, but the ambience and the sensitivities were all wrong. The main factor in my decision was that Mark and his team wouldn't be able to handle the smell. I think this was surely the right decision, as years later, one morning in 1997, Paul Holmes had flown down to film an item on conditions in New Zealand mortuaries. I was highly impressed with his energy, tight timetabling and absolute, natural friendliness.

He noticed the Latin inscription above the door: *Haec docebit ultra vivens mortua in ianuis.*

'What does that mean?' he held the microphone towards me.

'Beyond these doors, the dead teach the living,' I translated.

'Very erudite indeed. Let's go in.'

In less than five seconds, he was coughing into the back of his hand.

'What's that bloody awful smell?'

'That's nothing, really. It's not bad at all today. That's just the background smell of death. It's always here. We don't notice it.'

'How can you *not* notice it?'

'We do notice it when we get people here, say, after weeks in the river. They smell quite swampy. Now that's a smell to remember. But this, this is just low-level background normal.'

He grimaced. 'Smells like rancid fat to me, only worse. And those ghastly big steel doors? What are they? They look like Auschwitz or something.'

'Those are the fridges we store the dead in. Before we autopsy them,' I explained.

Paul became used to the smell after a few minutes and his tour and interview, which screened that evening, were quite enjoyable.

Most people notice the smell in the mortuary. It's not bad, just different. We are born with 100 per cent of the DNA in our body being ours, but soon after death, nearly 100 per cent of our DNA belongs to bacteria. In middle age, 70 per cent of the DNA we carry is bacteria and only 30 per cent is ours. Bacterial decay and bacterial dominance is part of life, and especially part of death. It has its own season and its own aroma.

* * *

Instead of the mortuary, we took Mark to the lab.

'This looks right,' Mark said, pointing at our advanced, multi-channel chemistry analyser. 'This is what I want as background.'

'But it's nothing to do with me at all. This is a biochemistry analyser. It has nothing to do with my job or post-mortems,' I pointed out.

'Don't worry yourself about that. But can you also put on a white coat?'

A white labcoat was rustled up for me. We hadn't worn white coats for a decade or more, but if that's what they wanted, I would happily oblige.

* * *

'I'm here in the medical laboratory talking to Dr Cynric Temple-Camp, the actual pathologist who did the autopsies on the Mezzatestas. Good morning, Doctor. Now I suppose that you really are an expert in, well, death?'

'Yes, I've certainly see my share of death over the years.'

Mark outlined the problem. Simultaneous deaths are a recognised problem and in the absence of any indication to the contrary, the law determines that the oldest dies first and the youngest last. That can change the outcome of an inheritance. Michael Mezzatesta was four years older than his wife so, according to the law, he died first and Diane inherited his property. The only way in which Michael Mezzatesta's brother could inherit was to establish that Diane died before her husband, by whatever slender margin.

The facts were straightforward. The Mezzatestas and their friend died in a head-on collision with a petrol tanker out on the State Highway 3. They had a rental car from Auckland and were driving through the night to get to their holiday destination in Marton. The driver of the truck reported that it was near dawn, 6.30 a.m., but with a reasonable amount of light, when the car drifted slowly across the midline and right under the front of his truck.

The friend was driving. Diane was beside him in the front seat, Michael in the back.

'And Doctor, you were able to identify them?'

'Not easily, no. They were so injured that they would be unsuitable for a visual identification. I mean, both vehicles were probably doing 100 kilometres per hour. And the car was dragged under the tanker for 50 metres. It was a large, fully laden petrol tanker, you see.'

'So they were identified how? Did you use DNA?'

'Not easily available then. We have a disaster identification process using dental records, which is pretty good. We managed to work out fairly well who was who. And also the truck driver's evidence helped a bit.'

'What did he say?'

'He looked down through the car windscreen a fraction of a second before they hit. He confirmed that there was a man

Accidents, Accidents, Accidents

and a woman in front, the man driving. He was wearing a red checked shirt. I was able to recover some of the shirt that was worn by the driver from the bits of body. The trucker said he thought they were both asleep as they showed no reaction right up to the second of impact. The coroner thought that this explanation sounded very reasonable.'

'The problem we are investigating is one of fair inheritance to the families. Can you help us with this one, Doctor?'

'Surely that's a matter for the lawyers, isn't it?'

'They seem to be finding it all a little perplexing. This is why Hinch is investigating.'

Mark focused on what the Australians needed to know. The biochemistry analyser chuntered quietly alongside, mechanically marching soldierly racks of ruby-red blood tubes past us.

Mark went on. 'As Diane was in the front seat surely she would die first? Michael would die later in the back seat, wouldn't he? If Diane is already dead, then the estate goes to Michael's brother, doesn't it? Michael is arguably still alive in the back seat at that instant even if it is only for a fraction of a second longer. Does that make sense?'

'Sounds messy, but I follow the argument so far.'

'Well, what do you think?'

'I think you need King Solomon, not a pathologist.'

'We might have to see if we can get an interview with him. Do you have his number?' We both smiled. 'But seriously, what do you think?'

'I think that the force that kills you is the massive deceleration at the instant of the impact. In head-on impacts

The Cause of Death

like this, the common injury is the heart gets ripped off the aorta. And all the blood then gushes out in seconds into your chest cavity. And you die.'

'Can you explain how that works?'

'Yes it's quite simple. The aorta is firmly attached to the back of the chest and the heart hangs freely off it like a pear in a tree. In a head-on collision, the heart instantly swings massively from going forward at 100 kilometres per hour to going backwards at 50 kilometres per hour and this just rips it off at the root. The aorta tears like tissue paper.'

I made a tearing apart gesture with my hands. The cameraman panned in closely, focusing in on them.

'And that happens at exactly the same time to everyone, no matter whether they're sitting in the front or back. I reckon they all died simultaneously, but hey, I'm just a pathologist and that's a pathological view. The lawyers will no doubt have their own methods of determining events.'

'And did the Mezzatestas both have these aortic injuries?'

'Yes, all three occupants did.'

And afterwards, I added in an aside, that this accident was the pity of life, because it need never have happened. They had already passed their turnoff to Marton. They must have been tired and just missed the sign. So they were already several kilometres past their destination when they met their destiny in the form of the truck.

* * *

Accidents, Accidents, Accidents

No-one knows when or if they have an appointment in the mortuary, but they very well may end up keeping one. Nothing is surer than dying: only the timing and the manner of death is unknown. Death is very often a surprise. I always wonder in this sort of case who deals with the Mezzatestas' apartment or house back in Melbourne. Who clears their post and tidies away the accumulation of two lives? What about their dog at the kennels? It is always my last thought when we head off on holiday. Who will look after things if we do not return? Perhaps humans are fortunate that our own, individual deaths are so unimaginable to us. Maybe that is what allows us to carry on.

CHAPTER 14

Questionable Evidence?

We place a very great deal of faith in the wisdom of the justice system, and the ability of the court system to deliver reasonable, impartial decisions. Sometimes that faith seems misplaced. I sat open-mouthed in the Privy Council in London, once, listening to the Law Lords declaring that serving soldiers in Afghanistan and Iraq could sue the British Army for failing to provide a safe work environment when they were on the battlefield. But that, I think, was one of those exceptions that proves the rule.

One Sunday morning, I found myself at work on what was supposed to be my day off. I was performing an autopsy on a 68-year-old man. He had apparently lost his temper with his neighbour's children who had a habit of climbing his wall to retrieve their football, trampling his flower beds and then fleeing before his purple rage. It seems his rage may have been the most exciting part of their game. Perhaps it was even the objective of it.

Questionable Evidence?

This time, he caught one of the kids by the scruff and had given him a good shake. The boy squealed to the heavens and his mother flew out of her house, hurling a yard broom as well as a torrent of foul abuse and threats at the man. The broom missed but the abuse didn't.

'Right! That's it! I'm going directly to the police, right now!' he yelled and off he strode. A hundred or so metres down the road, he fell over flat on his face dead from a heart attack. In hitting the pavement he split his nose and bled out a significant pool of blood around his head.

The police got a rather garbled version of events from other neighbours, and the children's mother was promptly arrested. The evidence the police received was questionable. Unfortunately the mother made matters worse by resisting arrest and vociferously abusing the police. She had a rather colourful turn of phrase and continued her tirade against the magistrate, who immediately ordered her to be detained over the weekend and to reappear before him on Monday, after she'd time to reconsider her behaviour.

I was asked to help by an officer from youth protection, who had found there was no-one home to look after the arrested woman's three children. So there I was in the morgue out of hours, seeing what I could do to ease frazzled tempers and restore some sanity to the situation by getting the mother back to her children. The deceased clearly had seriously diseased coronary arteries. His rage had released too much adrenaline, causing his arteries to go into spasm. That was enough to cut off the blood flow to his already damaged heart and he had dropped dead from a massive heart attack.

The Cause of Death

The cut on his nose had occurred after death and was caused by falling to the pavement.

The police were pragmatic: upon hearing this information, they arranged for the woman's release. She duly returned to her children.

I was then able to escape for a quiet Sunday afternoon siesta with the *Sunday Star Times*.

* * *

The quality of evidence was to the fore when, in 2013, Mark Lundy was back in my professional life once again. My evidence presented at his trial was now being called questionable. I was told that an appeal had been lodged with the Privy Council and was to be heard in London. Part of my evidence was in contention and would have to be answered.

I was flabbergasted. Surely, there could be nothing that could trump Rod Miller's superb, unequivocal demonstration of brain matter on the shirt?

I learned there was. Professor Philip Sheard felt he had done just that.

'Who?' I asked.

I thought I knew everyone working in forensic pathology in New Zealand, but it turned out that he wasn't a pathologist. He came from Otago Medical School's physiology department. Apparently he had declared Rod Miller's photographs, his methodology, his evidence in court, as well as the article that Rod, myself and others published in the *Forensic Pathology* journal, to be highly questionable

Questionable Evidence?

scientifically and with serious ramifications for Lundy's conviction.

I learned that an appeal had been lodged with the Privy Council saying there had been a miscarriage of justice based on poorly conducted and informed science. Amongst other grounds of appeal, there were two pathological areas in question. Professor Sheard's research denied the presence of brain tissue on Mark Lundy's shirt and believed he had scientific reasons to support this view. Separately a number of other experts disputed the opinion that was given to the trial on the timing of Christine's and Amber's deaths, on the grounds that gastric emptying was an unreliable method of determining it.

I was reeling at this information and quite distressed by it.

A few years before, I had been interviewed by a journalist who had written an article entitled: 'Dead men do tell tales' in which I was quoted as saying the discovery of brain in the Lundy case was a superb example of good science. I stood and stand by that statement. But here, 11 years on from his conviction, the Privy Council was being told that our science was bad and that Lundy may have been wrongfully convicted. Eleven years is a big chunk of someone's life. I hoped we hadn't made a terrible mistake.

I picked up Professor Sheard's manuscript and flicked through. At first glance, it was hugely impressive. It was beautifully prepared with dozens of colour photos. There were many pages of text as well as an avalanche of supporting scientific references.

My heart sank. Was it really possible that we had got something fundamentally wrong?

I shook my head and made myself put it aside. I had a load of surgical cases that needed reporting. I decided I would spend the weekend reading the new evidence.

* * *

Cameron Mander and Annabel Markham were the Crown counsel who would present the case to the Law Lords in London. I found them both impressive and knowledgeable, and affable with it.

'Why are you getting me to present evidence? You could get anyone in the world, surely?' I asked.

There were telephone discussions, emails and affidavits for months before it became clear. The issues were complicated but were simple when distilled to their essence.

'Tell us in a nutshell what Professor Sheard is saying?' I was asked.

'Well, simply put, he's saying the method used to show brain hasn't done so. He reckons Rod Miller's results weren't interpretable, that they were uncontrolled and that his selection of photographs gave an inaccurate representation of the facts.'

'What do you think of those claims?'

'It's difficult to know where to begin. Professor Sheard's opinions look like an authoritative scientific argument on the face of it. But I think it completely fails on the pathological criteria that I understand.' I shook my head. 'In fact, I don't believe it's scientific at all. It says that Rod Miller's photographs were selectively presented to support a conclusion. I honestly think that's bullshit.'

Questionable Evidence?

'Unfortunately, the Law Lords won't like that wording,' I was told. 'Can you think of another way of putting it?'

I was nonplussed but fortunately Professor Allen Gown from Vancouver came to my aid. He said the report was intellectual gamesmanship and definitely not science.

That heartened me. Professor Gown was one of the most highly regarded experts in the world in the field of immunohistochemistry. If he agreed, then I knew, for sure, there couldn't have been a mistake in the original work.

Because in the end, although Professor Sheard had even me doubting myself, I couldn't agree with Sheard's report. I had re-examined all the original slides lifted from the shirt. There were striking and strong positive markers all showing the distinctive pattern of brain.

I took photographs of the brain tissue on these slides, and showed them to many pathologists and even to some medical students. None had any hesitation in identifying the tissue as brain. It just could not be anything else. So how on earth could there be doubt?

A critical part of Professor Sheard's argument was that the shirt tissue had to be compared with identically prepared brain and thus he thought Rod Miller's controls were invalid.

As I explained to the Crown Counsel, this was perplexing. We used an identical control system to diagnose dozens of cancer patients every month. On the basis of these diagnoses, they were started on life-altering chemotherapy or radiotherapy. It wasn't just us down here in provincial New Zealand: pathologists throughout the world were all doing exactly the same thing — everywhere, by the hundreds of thousands.

The Cause of Death

'So tell us, as simply as you can, what these controls mean.'

'On each slide, there are several small pieces of brain, lung, liver and so on to compare with the shirt tissue. Brain has a unique inner structure, which is what the tissue on Lundy's shirt shows. Skin can only ever look like skin, lung can only be lung, kidney is the same, and brain can only ever look like brain. And this was brain. Full stop. It's not much more complicated than that.'

I had learned that Professor Sheard was a research scientist, a physiologist specialising in neurophysiology, which included work with rat brains. He was apparently highly respected in his field.

As they say, what goes around comes around. Smiling, I told the lawyers that perhaps there was a divinity punishing me for my presumption in carrying out a test during the original trial using rat brains, with which I'd had little experience. Should I be critical of Professor Sheard?

I knew that Sheard's opinion must be wrong, but there was more bad news to come. A group of eminent pathologists from the United Kingdom, including from Oxford University, had come out supporting it. It was claimed the brain tissue should never have been stained since there were 59 days between the murder and finding the shirt stain. These new experts seemed to believe that any brain would have decayed beyond recognition in that time.

I thought that was just nonsense. The dried brain-matter was preserved within minutes of the murder and was still preserved 59 days later and will still be so 59 years from now. Once it's fixed, it is preserved pretty much forever.

Questionable Evidence?

All pathologists should know that. Professor Gown had even pointed out that tissue dried for thousands of years and extracted from Egyptian and Peruvian mummies has been tested using exactly the same techniques and it has worked perfectly well.

To me, it was a farce of Shakespearian proportions. I told Cameron and Annabel that I was looking forward to seeing my dissenting colleagues cross-examined in the Privy Council. I was looking forward to being cross-examined myself, for I was sure my evidence was sound and would surely prevail.

They explained that there was to be no cross-examination in London. Only the two opposing sets of lawyers were allowed to present the scientific and other evidence to the Law Lords, who would then question them about it. It was a pity, for I was sure that competent cross-examination would have shown the opposing affidavits to be fundamentally flawed.

I could see a problem at once, because neither set of lawyers could have any practical insight into the pathology. How then could the Law Lords be expected to decide between contradictory expert opinions, to distinguish between fact and fiction? Could Cameron and Annabel put everything across to the court second-hand?

I could see that they were relishing the challenge. I was confident we had the science on our side and that the opposing side's arguments, while carefully constructed, were patently wrong.

We would just have to wait and see what could be done in London.

The Cause of Death

'Will I be allowed to attend?' I asked.

The answer was yes.

I booked my tickets. Wild horses wouldn't keep me away. And besides, the Wimbledon tennis open was on around the same time. I might be able to fit in a match or two between sessions, if I was lucky.

CHAPTER 15

Victims of a Disaster

The flight was atrocious. I was making my way to New Plymouth for a conference. I held a private pilot's licence and I have often flown myself about the countryside. That morning, I had picked up *Echo Bravo Hotel*, a Piper Warrior, at the Aero Club in Palmerston North and had edged my way north. The Stratford Gap was clagged-in by cloud so I returned to Whanganui and followed the coast around to New Plymouth instead. All the same, the conditions were ferocious. I was ambushed by a treacherous burst of crosswind and a wing lifted abruptly as I touched down. It was a relief to get everything flat and level on the ground and taxi to the terminal. Not long afterwards, I learned that some of our conference delegates couldn't make it in because Air New Zealand had cancelled their flight to New Plymouth.

I well know the severe and sudden weather that periodically batters and cloaks New Zealand, as well as just how dangerous it can be. The air has to be treated with great respect, particularly because of the unforgiving terrain that lies beneath. When I returned to Palmerston North, the weather seemed, if it was possible, to have deteriorated since my flight north-west two days earlier. My bones were shaken as the little aircraft was tossed and hurled from turbulent peaks to terrifying troughs over and over again. I kept the engine throttled well back as I wallowed slowly southwards. There was dense and angry grey cloud shrouding the horizon and rain lashed my windscreen, streaming across my vision in rivulets.

That turbulent weekend, my mind turned inevitably to the most tragic air accident I was ever involved in investigating.

It was on the night of 12 May 1988, the same time of year, almost to the day that a light aircraft, *Echo Quebec Alpha*, encountered similar weather over the same part of the country while en route from Hamilton to Whanganui. It never arrived.

I remember how relieved I was to be in bed at home that night as the rain roared on the roof and the house shifted uneasily under the sudden punch of a buffet of wind.

The phone rang. I looked at the clock. I had been asleep barely an hour.

'Dr Temple-Camp? Police here.'

The line crackled in sympathy with the storm as I heard the bad news, the worst possible news. There had been a major aircraft accident.

'Oh no! Where?'

I shuddered.

All the aviation accidents I had seen were difficult to deal with. I learned it was a charter flight, a twin-engined

Victims of a Disaster

Piper Seneca belonging to Foxpine Air Charters inbound for Whanganui, with a pilot and eight passengers on board. They failed to keep to their flight plan ETA. Radar and radio contact had been lost just before 18.30 hours. It looked bad, very bad. I felt a thrill of dread and fear roll through me. Mainly fear.

'We're pretty sure they've come down in the Ahu Ahu Valley. They're not answering calls. It's a pretty inaccessible location and we don't reckon that there's any way we can get anybody out of there tonight. This storm has closed everything down. We have a rescue team and paramedics ready to go in at dawn tomorrow.'

'Okay.' I thought rapidly through the procedures. 'Unlikely to be any survivors, then. So, this is going to be a disaster victim identification process.'

We had no real plans in those days to deal with civil disasters. Often in planning for disasters, the pathologists are forgotten. But they are crucial to the process. There are always only a few pathologists to go around at the best of times, and in very serious situations, there may be hundreds — if not thousands — of bodies to be catalogued and identified.

That's what happened with the Boxing Day Tsunami in 2004, which claimed a vast toll throughout Indonesia and the landmasses bordering the Indian Ocean. Tens of thousands of dead lay everywhere but there wasn't anything like enough pathologists to deal with the numbers.

The policeman told me they were planning to use the grid system of recovery to map the bodies in this sad task. The system had been invented to help recover remains

The Cause of Death

from Flight 901, an Air New Zealand DC-10 airliner that flew straight and level into the slopes of Mount Erebus in Antarctica in November 1979, and was now the gold standard for disaster recovery operations world-wide. It is based on the grid that was used in correspondence chess matches before the days of the internet. It allowed the precise location of each body or body part at the accident site to be recorded.

Why, you may wonder, do we bother with this difficult and time-consuming process?

It is partly to help in the reassembly of as much of each body as is possible in order to return the deceased to their families. They can then bury their loved ones. Equally important is the significance of the distribution of body parts and injury patterns, because this can help create a picture of how events unfolded at the time of impact.

The pathologist is always the deceased's last advocate. We tell the last story that the dead have to tell the living.

'Everything's in hand,' the policeman said. 'We'll probably start uplifting the first bodies to you tomorrow afternoon. I'll contact you as soon as we've located the wreckage and know what the local situation at the crash site is. Sleep well, Doc.'

I didn't, of course.

I slept badly. I dreamed I was flying again, heaving and turning, propellers and wings fusing into molten shapes and all was chaotically unformed and decorated with migrainous yellow streaks. All around was a dark purple hue and, in my nightmare, I could smell vomit. I felt myself heaving, a gut-wrenching hurl, and I knew this wasn't a dream. I sat up abruptly, retching, with burning fluid clawing in my throat as I choked on the raw taste of bile.

After that, I lay tautly awake knowing I had to scrape together sufficient courage to meet the horror of the task ahead. It was always the same at the start of any accident case. The waiting beforehand was the worst part. I have sometimes wondered if there's such a thing as a pre-traumatic stress disorder. I've often found that when my work was over and done with, it never seemed as bad as I'd anticipated. Usually I was fine and could set the tough assignment aside and sleep deeply and peacefully. It was my imagination beforehand that was a personal hell.

I'd had experience of air crashes, but that didn't make it any easier. It only meant that I knew what was lying out there on that cloud-enveloped, wet and weeping mountain.

* * *

It will have been a surreal scene. The dark, drenched figures of the police officers will have picked their way slowly across the slippery mountainside, carefully and intently studying the ground. The whole area will have been enveloped in a mesh of tapes, something like a giant spiders' web trapping the tragedy against the mountain side. The searchers will have dragged themselves from tape to tape, from square to square in the grid, while all around them will have been the scattered confetti of tortured and strained fragments of aluminium, the body of the aircraft broken into twisted chips by the unimaginable impact. Some fragments would have been recognisably painted, cream or red or blue or green, but many would have been shiny and metallic, all trace of colour scoured off by the impact. There might have been a length of a wing, perhaps, twisted grotesquely around a tree trunk, or a major portion of a mud-encrusted engine lying nearby, mottled with leaves, its twisted propeller still attached. Nothing much else will have been easily recognizable.

Fractured splintered branches would hang off the trees above. Some would bear weeping wounds, bark and wood torn away, with sap oozing to coat the scars. Across this slope and over all this activity, the rain would be falling, incessantly, cold and without vitality.

* * *

The waiting dragged on. They didn't uplift the bodies by the next afternoon, Friday the 13th, or even the next day, so difficult was their recovery. Each day, the investigation team had to hike through the bush, up the mountain slope. The way up was hard yakka, step by breathless step through the bush and across scree falls streaking the mountain. Then each night, they would make the steep descent after a long and weary day working at an almost impossible angle, collecting and marking every shred of tissue. It took the police search and rescue team three full days to complete the recovery.

The first body bags arrived on Sunday at midday, and we started work.

I looked down at them in the forecourt of the mortuary. Some body bags were big. Most were small. All were carefully labelled with grid number, time and date, and who found them. It was all meticulous evidence, recorded piece by bloody piece. Visitors to the scene in later years found toys and possessions that they claimed had been missed, and were critical of the team's efforts. But I can vouch for the fact that there was no carelessness. They were thorough, competent and professional. I believe those items had been hurled up into trees and bushes by the impact and were dislodged later by wind and had fallen to ground.

I had gone down to the mortuary early to begin preparations for the disaster victim identification process. We had only four mortuary tables, which was a problem, as nine bodies had to be reconstructed. We learned there were six adults, two children and an infant on board. It was as if we had nine different jigsaw puzzles mixed together and we had to reassemble them all from one pile of pieces.

But now the parts no longer fitted together. Also, some of the parts were missing, vaporised on impact or lost forever somewhere on that mountainside.

'Bruce,' I said to the head mortuary assistant. 'I want you to set up five separate tarpaulins as well as the tables. How about two in the loading foyer in front of the fridges and three in the ambulance bay?'

We were conveniently located next to the ambulance bay, sealed off from the road by large roller doors. All mortuaries are traditionally placed in the deepest bowels of the hospital in the basement — not to sweep away and hide the dead, but rather because access is needed for ambulances and hearses to discharge their tragic loads in private.

'Nah.' Bruce grimaced and shook his grey head dismissively. 'I reckon we can do four on the tables, and I can fit all five tarps in the ambulance bay easy. The body bags we'll pile in front of the fridges and work through them one by one, putting the pieces in the right places. Reckon that would be best.'

'Okay,' I agreed. 'Label the stations one to nine.'

The plan was to reassemble each jigsaw in its own station, one station per body.

There were four pathologists available to do the reconstruction. Roy Darby was the local head of pathology and there was my colleague James and there was me. Ash, the chemical pathologist who normally spent his time analysing laboratory samples, was summonsed to help, in view of the gravity and complexity of the task.

The first part was pretty straightforward.

There was one body, a woman, who was largely intact. Of course, there were the usual multiple fractures, bruises, contusions and lacerations which were familiar to me from my work with accidents. Her clothes were torn and muddied — a dark red jacket, white jersey, black skirt — and her shoes were missing. She was, however, easily identifiable. She was a well-built, olive-skinned woman with dark hair, bright red lipstick and toenails and fingernails carefully painted to match. She would have been about mid-forties, I estimated. She had been seated in the single seat in the rear of the cabin.

For the rest, we were able to identify major portions of torso and we placed one in each station, one for each known passenger. That was our starting point around which we had to build each reconstruction.

The indefatigable police recovery team came off the mountain estimating that they had made a better than 50 per cent recovery. That would be an outstanding result.

They presented us with a whiteboard on which was marked a grid with the main impact site denoted by a red X. It represented a clinical and sanitised analytical picture with little resemblance to the noxious, meaty and dank hecatomb on the side of that dreadful mountain.

* * *

As each body part was positively identified, it was reunited with the appropriate body at the designated mortuary station. The grid number, where the part had been found, was then written on the whiteboard under the victim's name. We each had a police officer to act as a scribe, who also had the responsibility of keeping the whiteboard up to date, assigning each identified piece to its grid and body. The grid numbers built up on the board: 2/4/1, 3/6/8, 2/4/10, 3/6/5. Little by little, as the fragments were identified we were able to build up a picture of exactly where each body had spread on impact. As the bigger picture came into focus, it showed carnage. There were parts flung violently to all points of the compass and beyond. It was more like an explosion than an impact.

All this effort might not be important in the end. But we would only know that afterwards, when the results had been

The Cause of Death

analysed by the crash investigators. Our job was to persist and get it right.

* * *

I've always thought it would be a good idea to place a colour photograph of each victim at their station. This would have helped us, because we were using skin colours and hair tints to identify body parts. But equally important, we should have been reminded at all times that these were real people, no longer living, but were our patients to whom we owed a duty of care and compassion.

I chose to work on the pilot. He had proved relatively easy to identify. He had a reddish beard as well as a lightly freckled, pale skin. The fine hairs on his skin struck a reddish gold light when looked at on an angle. As I went through the tissue bags, it was easy to spot his distinctive skin, to retrieve it together with its attached tissue and begin the process of restitution. I had begun with his largest piece, which was part of the upper chest. I worked through this cavity searching for the heart and I found a map plastered against his spinal column. A glance told me that this was his flight plan. I could picture him with it folded on his knee for easy reference as he fought to control his aircraft through those final seconds.

There were shreds of clothing intimately mixed with the fragments of tissue as well as ample leaf mould, all well salted with a condiment of mountain mud. I came to recognise a dark blue material that I guessed was his shirt, as well as fragments of cream-coloured shorts, a dark green Parka leaking fluffy padding as well as a liberal scattering of zipper teeth.

But otherwise, there was surprisingly little clothing to find. They had been shredded by the impact.

We almost had them right first time, and we had only to do a little rearranging before we were happy we had the passengers identified. And then it was a matter of assigning the multiple fragments back to their owners.

But of the infant who was supposed to have been aboard, there was absolutely no sign — nothing whatever on which to start building. His tarpaulin lay on the floor appealing mutely, dry, unstained and waiting.

We identified the second torso I worked on as one of the woman passengers because of her bone structure and build. There were no obvious, distinctive features by which to confirm who she was. Her skin was light and unblemished, perhaps, I thought, a trifle paler than the skin on any of the other bodies, but that was very subjective. I was working deep within the pelvic cavity when I found a strange thing.

Enveloped within the bony blades of the pelvis and forming a hard bridge across to the lumbar spine was a mass of unidentifiable tissue. It was firmly attached, wedged deep within the cavity.

What on earth is this? I was puzzled. It didn't look like any anatomical organ that I could recognise. Could it be a tumour? An unknown cancer revealed only by death and an accidental evisceration?

I gradually prised the mass free from the protective grip of the pelvic bones. It resisted, then came out suddenly and with a moist, wrenching sound.

I looked. We all looked.

Suddenly I recognised it.

'It's the infant!' I said. 'It's the missing infant.'

Everyone gathered around looking in sorrowful fascination.

'I don't know whether this woman is the boy's mother. Maybe he was sitting on her lap at impact. I should have thought of that before.'

A cloak of sadness fell across the mortuary, and the work stopped. All conversation died away.

In death, the child and the women were closely knit. In a way it was comforting to know they were together.

It was a profound and sombre moment. We stood in silence for a long while, just looking.

For some time after this terrible discovery, the mortuary was quiet with everyone lost in their own thoughts.

* * *

It took us two full days and it wasn't until 11 o'clock on the morning of the third day that we were pretty well done. All the identifiable parts had been assigned and there were only smaller, unidentifiable flecks of tissue remaining that we couldn't assign to any of the passengers.

The bodies were bagged and in the freezers awaiting release by the Coroner. The police had gone apart from the officer in charge.

Victims of a Disaster

'Coming to lunch, Doc?' the OC asked. 'I figure the boys need a wind down, a bit of R & R. Police shout. We've booked a table for 25 up at Cobb & Co for noon. Reckon we deserve a few beers and a bit of relaxation.'

'Okay, thanks. I'll be there.'

I felt my spirits lift. Now that the worst part of the work was done, I guess I got a second wind, because I found I was no longer tired. And to my surprise, I was starving. Days of living on plates of sandwiches from the hospital cafeteria meant I could do with a good meal and a beer.

I was at the mortuary bench studying a floret of five ribs with their web of intercostal muscles. As hard as I'd tried, I couldn't find a place for them in any of the nine bodies. It irked me, because it was the largest unassigned piece of body left. I thought there had to be a clue, if I could look and think hard enough.

Certainly they were from an adult. That only eliminated the children and the infant. Certainly they were from the left side. That could be any one of the adults. All were deficient in ribs, particularly from the left side.

I picked up the ribs and stared at them blankly. I studied them and pushed them apart with my hands. Splayed out in my hands they stayed stubbornly mute to me. But there was unmistakeably the sweetish smell of early decomposition.

The ends of the ribs as I studied them were cleanly severed cut, as though a surgeon had performed the cut — a surgeon, or a butcher.

Their smell was suddenly nauseating, and coagulated in that precise spot in my throat where smell suddenly turns into taste.

The Cause of Death

'Bloody ribs!' I thought and spat into the sink. I put the tissue back into the fridge and left to catch up with the team for lunch.

* * *

Cobb & Co was warm with thick, oily air, delicious to breathe, and an aroma that stimulated a hunger that only solid food could erase. The restaurant was full. Along one wall was a long table set up for us. Loud and excited policemen, flushed with the promise of the aroma, the warmth and the rising pleasure of beer, were happily chatting, calling out to one another, chaffing, joking and laughing. It was as though a cork had been drawn on a long pent-up maestrom of emotion. We were a convivial and contented group.

I sat down and a pint glass of beer was pushed into my hand.

Tui beer. The best.

I drank a long, deep draught. 'God, I needed that. Especially after this week.'

'Good on you, Doc.' A policeman raised his glass to me. 'Drink up. You're a bit behind the rest of us already!'

I looked round the table. Strong, honest faces, sons of farmers, mostly, men who had worked sheep hard across the ranges. Policemen. They were the salt of the earth. I couldn't think of a finer place to be at this time, or finer men to be with.

The waitress placed a platter in front of me. Other platters landed thudding beneath their steaming loads on either side, across the table, all around me. A cohort of waitresses had descended upon us, placing our food before us simultaneously, smiling happily as the men called out to them.

I looked down.

Ribs.

I caught my breath.

They had ordered ribs. Pork spare ribs. Dozens of them. The sawn ends oozing fat, pointing at the ceiling, the ribs themselves glistening with marinade.

My stomach heaved involuntarily at the sight of them, but I caught it in time.

Oh God. Not ribs please! Any other day, but not today. Not after all this!

Fries on the side with bloody bowls of tomato sauce as well.

My stomach fought and lost the battle. A wave of nauseous disgust flooded my brain. It was too much. I got up and ran outside leaving them there, watching me go, their mouths open in astonishment. It was the only occasion on which I ever just lost it.

* * *

The inquest for the nine victims of the Ahu Ahu Valley plane crash was held in Whanganui. The Coroner, Colin Riddert, agreed that I could give evidence on behalf of all four pathologists to avoid repetition and to make the flow of evidence smoother. A benchful of lawyers representing the charter company was present, as well as people from the company that maintained the Seneca, plus the relatives of the victims and other interested parties.

The court was packed. This was unusual. Normally there would be only the coroner, myself, a few relatives and one policeman. We had only two useful pieces of pathological evidence to come from our autopsies. This was always going to be a tricky case, with the main question in my mind being: would our evidence be of any help?

The first problem was that of aircraft loading — or more specifically, overloading. All aircraft have a maximum take-off and landing weight, laid down by the designers and manufacturers. But that's not enough. The passengers have to be seated and the luggage distributed so that the centre of gravity of the plane lies inside carefully calculated limits. That's why on long-haul international flights, if you've been lucky enough to score a bank of empty seats on which to sleep, the cabin staff will always ask you to return to your allocated seat for landing. The critical balances are that fine.

Unbalance the aircraft by going outside these limits and the plane can become uncontrollable very quickly, especially in bad weather. A coroner thought a shifting balance point is what happened in 2010 where nine people died in a crash on the take-off of their aeroplane at Fox Glacier. It was thought the shifting weight of a skydiver who accidently slid backwards towards the open door as the plane climbed on take-off was enough to throw the whole aircraft out of kilter.

The inquest heard that four additional passengers had boarded the Seneca in Hamilton and the pilot couldn't cram

Victims of a Disaster

their luggage into the already full lockers. Their luggage was placed between the passenger seats in the rear of the cabin.

It was the makings of a disaster.

Our input to this part of the investigation was largely guesswork and was based on estimating the post-mortem weights of the individual passengers in order to calculate their contribution to the overall centre of gravity problem. There was an argument that as two of the passengers were children and one was an infant, the balance may have been better than it looked at first glance.

The lawyers were dogged in trying to pin us down to precise weights for the individual passengers we had autopsied.

'Surely that's simple, Doctor?' one lawyer asked, sounding almost contemptuous. 'Surely you can weigh the bodies? Is that not routine? Why is the weight not recorded in some of your reports?'

This was awkward. The answer was simple, of course. The bodies were fragmented, the retrieval was maybe of only 50 per cent of the total tissue mass of all of the passengers, and who could lay their hand on their heart and swear we'd correctly assigned all of it? I felt my mouth full of dry cotton as I looked up at the public gallery. There sat the relatives, sombre and grey. Already there had been the sound of sobbing. A woman, grey-haired with shoulders hunched, left the court with her hobbling husband shepherding her awkwardly from behind.

How could I explain to this lawyer just what we had had to do, little though it was, just to piece these people together again so there was something to go home? Had he ever even seen a dead body?

This particular evidence didn't matter anyway, but that has never stopped lawyers asking. For the Court of Inquiry was able to determine that the Seneca was unbalanced. Two adult passengers and their luggage should not have been aboard.

The second question was much more interesting, from my point of view, both as a pilot and as a naturally curious human being. At the moment of impact, the aircraft had its wheels and flaps down, which is the normal set-up to land. Pilots will tell you that is only ever done when in the final landing pattern at the airport, so why this configuration 20 nautical miles away to the north of the airport?

Flying on instruments is great. It is well-established and is safely performed a hundred thousand times each day. One instrument used to create this miracle is the non-directional beacon, which is a rather imprecise name for a very precise instrument. It is a wonderful device to use to guide you home when blinded by awful weather.

It has some weaknesses, though. Its radio waves can be reflected back by the ionosphere at sunset. Mountains and cliffs can cause anomalous readings as well, and electrical storms can cause the Automatic Direction Finder (ADF) needle to deflect towards the activity.

Witnesses on the ground had seen the aircraft come out of cloud and turn west and adopt an approach similar to that used coming into Whanganui Airport. It was thought that some or all of these weaknesses may have given the pilot

Victims of a Disaster

a false signal, misleading him to believe he was over the Whanganui airport and that he should begin his descent to land in the wrong place.

It all sounded quite plausible.

The alternative was that a heavily overladen aircraft, climbing and diving wildly in severe turbulence, with speeds swinging between excessive and stalling, was out of control. The cabin would be a maelstrom of emotions, with terrified passengers, including young children, an infant in arms and loose baggage. The pilot may have lowered flaps and wheels to increase drag in order to reduce the variations in speed.

If that were the case, at that point, it was over. The aircraft entered a spiral dive and at 18.37 hours hit the steeply wooded hillside of the valley 19 nautical miles north of Whanganui.

Which scenario was right? Did our findings support one or the other?

It is difficult to deduce with complete certainty what occurred in the last seconds from the injuries we had documented. We had discussed this at some length and thought that descending straight and level into the ground would spread the wreckage and victims, at the moment of impact, in a line along the aircraft's flight path. In level terrain, the debris would be spread over a hundred metres or more, but of course impact with the steep side of the mountain might change everything. We didn't think the pattern of injuries substantially supported that possibility.

What if it dived out of control, no longer flying, but auguring straight into the ground?

The Cause of Death

We thought the wreckage and bodies would be in a relatively confined area. Much of the wreckage might be buried. The degree of breakup would be more massive and the severity and degree of dismemberment of the victims much greater — exactly as we had found.

The pilot and seven of the passengers all showed similar injuries. The bodies were diced into multiple pieces, showing evidence of a razor-like dicing rather than the crushing fragmented destruction with which we are so familiar with in high-speed vehicle accidents. Most of this grisly debris was flung in an arc up and down the slope from the impact site, as we had seen marked on the grid of the whiteboard in the mortuary.

The pathologists all thought that the death was instantaneous on impact but then an engine propeller had been crushed into the cabin, whirling and dicing and hurling the bodies widely across the slope. That is what the mapping told us. There was one intact body, although obviously still with the multiple injuries expected in such a high-speed accident. We deduced that because she was seated at the rear, the propeller had missed her.

I had read all the reports and had prepared to present our combined evidence. But no-one asked specifically about the interpretation of the pattern of injuries, and being new to the New Zealand system I was unsure whether it was my place to volunteer it unasked. I guessed that the court was overwhelmed by the enormity of the disaster and this question did not occur to any of the legal advocates present whose main focus was on the more narrow issue of the passengers' weights.

Victims of a Disaster

It made no difference in the end. The Court of Inquiry eventually discounted the false beacon theory and found the sequence of events to be exactly as we had deduced from our findings.

* * *

I have always enjoyed the tough professional challenge of investigating deaths in air crashes and have always volunteered for them. I think being a pilot and having an aviation background adds another perspective. Most pilots are seriously interested in the cause of crashes. After all, as the macabre joke runs, they know the pilot is always the first to arrive at the scene of an accident!

The challenge in these autopsies is threefold. The first is to check for a medical condition in the pilot and carry out toxicology tests looking for alcohol or drugs that could have resulted in a sudden loss of consciousness. Positive drug or alcohol tests are very rare and it is uncommon to find an unrecognised medical condition, since pilots have regular and rigorous medical checks to maintain their licences. As I learned to do way back when in Rhodesia, we also look for fractures to hands and feet that are inflicted by the aircraft's controls during impact with the ground. If these specific injuries are present, it means the pilot was conscious and trying to control the aircraft on impact.

Second is to look at the overall pattern of injuries to see what the directional forces were on impact, much as we did in the Ahu Ahu disaster. Finally, we check for seatbelt and harness injuries to confirm the correct restraint was in place. That's about it.

It sounds simple, but it usually takes all day, often longer than complicated heart surgery. And for all that, our findings can sometime be misleading.

It was my sombre duty to examine the body of my good friend Guy Lawton and his two young sons, Matthew and Samuel, after an air accident. Guy was an outstanding oral and maxillofacial surgeon at Palmerston North and an avid pilot. On a flight home to Paraparaumu one night, his twin-engine Piper Navajo, *Tango Zulu Charlie*, had an engine failure and he turned back to Feilding aerodrome. Unfortunately, a strong tailwind had sprang up. As Guy climbed away to make a second approach, the plane stalled and spun into the ground.

People often ask how I can perform autopsies on my friends.

I see it as an honour. They have come under my care and I will look after them professionally and with compassion as any doctor would. So it was with a heavy heart but great determination that I set to work on Guy.

He had been at a party that night but his blood alcohol was zero. Guy was a flamboyant man, full of a zest for life, but he would never drink and fly: I hardly needed to see the test results to know that for sure.

His background medical condition did not suggest anything amiss, although there were some lymph glands in his chest that looked a little enlarged to me. Investigation showed the glands contained granulomas. Guy had unrecognised sarcoidosis, which is a generalised disease of the body. No-one knows the cause, but small clumps of white blood cells called macrophages settle in aggregates or granulomas, mainly in the lung and lymph glands, but also the skin, salivary glands, liver, spleen and sometimes, unfortunately, in the heart.

Its significance is that if there is cardiac sarcoid, these granulomas can cause scarring and arrhythmias. That is, it causes irregularities of heartbeat and these can, of course, cause sudden incapacitation and death. This occurs in 40 per cent of patients with sarcoid, according to the medical textbooks. But sarcoid is more common than we think. The Royal Air Force carried out an investigation of their personnel and found that it was four times more common than formerly believed, and appeared to have little effect generally and none whatsoever on their pilots. The textbooks are certainly overstating the case.

Guy's lungs and heart were also involved with the sarcoid but there was no evidence that the disease was implicated in causing the crash. While his disease had raised a flag, it was quite correctly judged irrelevant in this case. All the other circumstances told a different and compelling story. I was honoured to be able to look after Guy, Matthew and Samuel that day.

Farewell, my friend.

CHAPTER 16

Dangerous Elements

'Doctor, I think you had better come down to the mortuary.'

I had 23 difficult biopsies to examine, and time was running out. Patients would be returning to clinics or, worse, lying in the wards waiting for me to make up my mind so they could get on with their lives or with getting the treatment they needed.

A senior registrar was on duty in the mortuary and I had been hoping for at least a couple of uninterrupted hours with my diagnostic problems. There was nothing she couldn't handle. She had dealt with suicide, gunshot wounds, traffic accidents and even the occasional mound of decomposed flesh and bone. I trusted her judgement completely.

I hurried down to the mortuary. Everyone was subdued. I turned to Pat, the mortuary assistant.

He shook his head slightly and looked at the ground before him. 'There're three kids in there.' Pat nodded towards the examination room. 'All drowned.'

'What happened?' I asked quietly.

'The families were having a picnic down at Totara Reserve. Kids were swimming, four of them from two families. Tea was ready so one of the fathers calls them out.' Pat angrily dashed tears from his eyes. His voice was cracking with emotion. I had never seen him like this before.

'The fucking cliff came down on top of them. In front of everyone.'

My eyes were wet too. I felt nauseous.

'So they were crushed by the rocks? How did they get the children out?'

'The fathers dived in and got the two boys out. The young girl got washed downstream.'

I suddenly wanted to be far away; wanted this to be over and for me to be somewhere else, in a safe time and place. I wasn't sure I could do this, but knew I had to.

I looked at Pat and the registrar. 'Let's go and do this. It's time these children went home.'

They were beautiful. I stopped and stared for a good long while. All three were unmarked. Drowned.

A picture from my childhood flashed into my mind. It was a picture from a beautifully illustrated *Treasure Casket* book, a brightly coloured illustration of Tom and the Water Babies. I had read and re-read the story as a boy. I was entranced by a picture in the book of two happy, smiling young girls floating effortlessly underwater in the river, their hair floating in the current, with Tom seated on the river-bed smiling up at them, while weeds waved in the flow.

The Cause of Death

'How can the Water Babies breathe?' I had wondered. 'How can they be so happy and smile like that underwater?'

But of course, they couldn't. Not in real life. No-one can breathe underwater. They would drown. That wondering child was now long gone and in his place stood a shocked pathologist confronted by three drowned children.

Two hours later, my examination was complete. My finding was not what I had expected. I sat quietly in my office and thought a long while.

I went to see Graham Hubbard, the Coroner, to discuss it.

'Graham, how are you, sir?' I shook his hand and sat in the chair opposite his desk. A messy pile of rolled legal files lay on the floor beside his chair, but his desk top was clear, immaculate.

'Very good to see you again, Doctor. Very good indeed. Now what am I to make of this tragic matter? The children swimming in the pool, and on whom the cliff fell.'

'Well, it's not quite that simple, Graham. The cliff didn't in fact fall directly onto them. It landed beside them, although it seems debris was thrown out horizontally after it hit the surface. They didn't drown, either, although it was the three in the deeper water who were caught. It is a bit more complex than that. And I think the findings are significant.'

'Explain your findings, please.'

'The information at first was that they had drowned. Everyone thought so, especially after it was clear that the cliffs hadn't actually landed on top of them. So what had happened? They could all swim well. To me, that was the puzzle. What I will say in court is that all three died of precisely the same pattern of injury. They all had fracture dislocations of their necks, and two also had fractures of the base of their skulls. These spinal dislocations would have caused instant death — without any suffering, I can say with certainty. They didn't die by drowning. Oddly, their other injuries were superficial, and not life-threatening.'

'And what are the implications of this observation?' said Graham.

'Impossible to know for sure. The public perception is that the cliff fell on them, but that doesn't appear to be the direct mechanism. They were all swimming at the time, heads above water, playing as kids do, yet they didn't drown. The fall was a short distance away, but it was a massive volume. It looks to me as if the fall has sent a shock wave through the water, like a riverine tsunami if you like. It was a racing tidal shock wave accelerating rapidly through the water. The result was inevitable. The shock wave travelled along the surface of the water and smashed the swimmers' heads, a sharp blow, savage enough to fracture their spines.'

We sat in silence for several minutes.

'They never had a chance, then, did they?'

'No. I suppose if you knew about the shock wave and if you recognised what was happening, you might dive. Dive below the surface, I mean. Divers beneath the surface of tsunamis at sea have come to the surface with no idea at all that anything's happened above. The tsunami is a surface phenomenon only.'

'Does it make any difference? Not to these poor children, I mean, but to the public?'

The Cause of Death

'Well, the council has put up signs that say BEWARE OF THE DANGER OF FALLING CLIFFS. That's true as far as it goes. But is that really useful? Will it stop lives being lost if there is another fall? I doubt it. Based on what I've seen, I guess the only message is if you swim in a river pool and the cliff drops, you may well be killed even if you're not actually under the fall. The shock wave of the slip hitting the water may well kill you even if you aren't hit by debris. So, now we've learned that at least, I think. But I have one further thing to say.'

Graham raised an eyebrow. 'Go on.'

'Even though I know about this danger, I'll keep swimming in those swimming holes below those cliffs, and below other cliffs in other rivers. It's part of our lives here in this country and, after all, we can't protect ourselves from absolutely every possible act of nature, can we? We live on islands shaken by earthquakes. These events are tragic but rare. Nature and the elements will always be unpredictable. Why should we stop swimming in rivers just because something bad might happen? Part of me thinks there is nothing much we can do to protect ourselves from nature. I reckon you've got more chance of being hit by a falling tree than by a falling cliff.'

I sadly gave the causes of death at the packed inquest.

* * *

One Monday evening I was watching the six o'clock news. The weather forecast followed.

'The Met Office has issued a heavy weather warning for the Lower North Island for this afternoon and evening. A

Dangerous Elements

low-pressure front is rapidly approaching from the southwest, and extreme high winds, rain and snow will follow. Gusts up to 200 kilometres per hour are expected in exposed places. Flooding is probable especially in low-lying areas. People are advised to move stock into more sheltered areas and to avoid unnecessary travel over this period. People are also advised to secure loose objects from the wind and to be aware of the danger of falling trees.'

Severe weather fronts are common in New Zealand and mostly we cope and get on with things. I was warm and comfortable and had a great book to read. I had just bought *My Sister's Keeper* by Jodi Picoult and was eager to get into it.

And this was no idle weather warning: hail rattled at the windows. The house shivered with the impact of the wind. At the height of it, strictly following Murphy's law, the phone rang.

'Evening, Doc. Pat here.'

'Patrick! What's up?'

'Just heard there's an SAR in the Tararuas.'

SAR. Search and Rescue. I winced. These rarely ended but one way, especially in extreme conditions such as these.

'What's happened?'

'A couple and their dogs went there for a tramp. Pretty experienced, but something must have happened. No sign of them. SAR teams have gone in tonight.'

Another slash of hail bruised the window panes.

'Bloody hell!' I said. 'This weather's not survivable, is it? The wind must be a hundred knots at least.'

The Cause of Death

'Yep. Gusting 200 k they say, and snowing. It's well below zero up there. We're looking for bodies for sure.'

Tuesday came. The weather had moderated, but it was still blowing a gale and freezing. There was no word from the mountains. Up there, men dressed in Antarctic clothing were pressing into the teeth of it, their weatherbeaten faces battered into expressionlessness, driven on by the ever fainter possibility of a live rescue.

Afternoon tea time arrived. I'd had one bite of a muffin and had not yet sipped my coffee in the hospital cafeteria, when Pat tapped me on the shoulder.

'They've recovered a body, the woman. The man has been choppered in with hypothermia. We're on. But finish your muffin first.'

The muffin had lost its appeal.

I heard the tragic story. The rain had swollen the Ohau River and the couple couldn't cross back to safety. They were experienced trampers and decided to head for the Waiohepu Hut for shelter. Unfortunately, this took them into the worst of the ferocious storm. A dog was lost. The woman slipped while crossing a river and injured her back. The wind repeatedly buffeted them to the ground. They forced their way on but just short of the hut, in winds of over 100 kilometres an hour, in driving rain and sub-zero temperatures, the woman could go no further. The man did everything to save her, did his heroic best, but it was too much to ask and she died of exposure.

* * *

Dangerous Elements

'So why does a person die of exposure, Doc?' The mortuary assistant was looking at me quizzically.

The autopsy had been unremarkable. As usual in cases of hypothermia, there was nothing to find, because death is caused by fibrillation of the heart, which leaves few signs.

The mortuary assistants have a difficult job. They download bodies from the fridges and wheel them into the mortuary. The bodies are then gently lifted onto the examination table so the autopsy can proceed. None of this is any different to a patient being wheeled into theatre for an urgent operation. We are always as careful with the dead as theatre staff are with the living.

The assistants also have to return all organs into the vacated body cavities and then cosmetically stitch up the skin before the bodies are returned to the deceased's families. The assistants have no part in the actual dissection to determine the cause of death, but they are always interested and we pathologists encourage them to ask questions. The more they know, the more interested they become and the better they are as technicians.

I always like to talk to the staff as I work.

'I'll tell you what it was like. The weather front came over, the temperature dropped nearly 30 degrees, the wind came up to 120 kilometres per hour. If you're in ordinary heavy-weather mountain gear, you've got maybe five minutes of conscious reasoning time left. In ten minutes you will be dead. The wind at those temperatures will strip every calorie of heat from you, even through your clothes, and you'll die. Even in Arctic gear, your survival is 20 minutes maximum unless you can find shelter. You'll die of exposure, like that!' I snapped my fingers in the air.

I explained that in hypothermia people reach a stage where their temperature control is totally lost and they sense cold as heat. Survivors say they felt boiling hot, and it is an agonising feeling. They can't help but strip off. It's common to find hypothermia victims hiding in a cave in the foetal position covered with bits of grass or leaves. It's called the 'Hide and Die' syndrome. We don't usually find much. The eyes are usually glazed with frost, but the fatal event is a final, massive electrical arrhythmia that stops the delivery of blood to the brain. At that point, you fall into a gentle, soft sleep. Except, of course, it's not sleep. It's death.

* * *

Pat greeted me at the mortuary door. 'A straightforward drowning on the table.'

'I hope it's not a child. I'm just not feeling up to that today.'

'Nah, a 72-year-old man. Out in his boat off a reef. Diving for paua. His son is in the viewing room with the body. He was on board at the time too, and wants to talk to you.'

'Okay. Bring him into the office. I'll talk to him before changing.'

The son was a big man, over a hundred kilograms, I guessed, and tall with it. He was clearly a farmhand by his clothing and boots. I introduced myself. His shake was crushing, a grip seasoned by years of hard labour.

'I'm sorry to hear about your dad. Can you tell me what happened?'

'We'd just anchored off a good paua spot. Dad dived down. He's been doing it for years — as long as I can remember, since I was a nipper. He'd just dived, when a fucking enormous wave came out of nowhere.'

I nodded. 'I've heard of these rogue waves. They're quite common along the coast. A couple of fishermen drowned off the rocks along there after being hit by one.'

'That'd be right. But it didn't break on us. The anchor rope was snagged on something and was too short so the boat couldn't rise. It just pulled us under. When I came up, the boat was upside down, but floating. I swam over and hung on. I couldn't see Dad anywhere so I called out. He was right there!'

A tear formed in his eye and he blinked it back.

'Right where?'

'Under the fucking boat! He called out. He was in the air-pocket underneath. He must have surfaced by chance under the boat, and he yelled out "What happened?" I mean, what are the chances?'

I nodded sympathetically.

'I shouted at him: "It's a fucking wave, Dad. Just dive down and come up on this side." I heard him say, "Okay".'

His tears flowed freely now. 'We're not surprised he didn't make it. He's pretty crook at the moment.'

Aha, I thought. He's probably gone diving with a dicky heart.

'What's been his problem then?' I said. 'Is it his ticker?'

'Nah. He got the liver cancer. Terminal, his doctor says. He goes for chemotherapy for it.'

Now that was odd. Chemotherapy for liver cancer is toxic, really very toxic. Your hair falls out, you vomit all the time and you feel pretty bad, like the worst dose of flu you could imagine. You wouldn't, generally speaking, be in the mood to go paua diving.

'Really? When did he finish his treatment?'

'He still goes for it. Been going for over a year now. Every second week he goes to hospital for treatment because it's terminal, you see.'

I didn't see, really. I didn't know of any treatment regime for liver cancer that was carried out like that.

'So we're okay with it all,' he was saying. 'The old man was terminal, so it wasn't a bad way to go. He would have liked that.'

* * *

The deceased's body was shorter than his son's but he was well-muscled and looked fit and strong. He didn't look a day over 50. There was none of the wasting that you'd expect with terminal cancer. What's more, he had a full head of hair, still a natural brown, no greying at all. That was unusual at 72, but it happens. It's unheard of in people who have been receiving chemo for a long time.

There was some lightly bloodstained froth around the nostrils. I often saw that in drownings.

I split his chest open.

Dangerous Elements

The lungs unexpectedly ballooned out of the chest cavity, massive and pink and spongy with a few darker flecks. They sprang out and actually joined, touching in the midline and totally obscuring the heart. The grooves of the ribs were etched deeply into their mass.

'Emphysema aquosum,' I breathed to myself.

'What's that?' Pat was standing close by and heard my whisper.

'Emphysema from drowning. Don't see it very often. In fact, this is only the third one I've seen out of dozens of drownings.'

'What's it from?'

'Apparently the victim gulps air in but doesn't or can't let it out again. So their lungs just keep inflating. Like blowing up a balloon. Except it can't pop because of the rib cage. That's why you can see the rib marks on the lung. But the thin air sac walls inside the lung, they pop all right. He would be different because the only air he breathed was in the pocket under the boat. Maybe that was under some pressure so his last lungful before diving would just keep expanding as he came up again. That would blow up and pop his lungs for sure.'

'So he drowned?'

'Probably. But I'll check to make sure.'

I inserted a large-bore needle through the thin skull bone above his eye socket into the ethmoid sinus hidden within the bones of the skull. I pulled back on the plunger and the syringe filled up with crystal-clear water. I drew out 25 millilitres. There was still more to come.

'Drowned for sure.' I gave the syringe to Pat. 'Take that up to the lab and ask them to measure the sodium level. Tell them to dilute about 500 times before testing.'

'And if they ask why?'

I smiled. 'They won't. But just so you know, it's seawater and salty. You could taste it as a shortcut, if you like.'

Pat shook his head vigorously as he held up the syringe, looking at the fluid in the light.

'How'd it get there?'

'If you breathe under water, the water will be sucked into your sinuses. It's got nowhere else to go. So a sinus full of water proves you tried to breathe under water and so drowned. If it's a dead body that's been dumped in water, the sinuses will be dry. And of course, if you drown in seawater, the sinuses are full of seawater. But if you drowned in the bath and then were dumped in the sea, the sinuses would be full of fresh water, which has no salt, and no sodium to measure. So go upstairs and get that sodium result and let's prove it's seawater while I do the dissection.'

His body was completely healthy. Like his looks, his internal body paralleled that of a 55-year-old. I could find no cancer anywhere.

* * *

I searched our database and all of the regional cancer services. I could find no trace of this man under treatment for liver or any other cancer anywhere in the country. I even tried the

Cancer Registry. They had no hits against any version of his name, NHI number or date of birth.

* * *

'I have a favour to ask.'

'What?' the policeman who had filled out the Pol-47 for this man's drowning sounded suspicious.

I told him about my findings and the lack of any cancer. 'The story just isn't right. I'm fairly sure there isn't anything criminal here, but something's not adding up. I don't think we need any formal investigation, but maybe you could have a look into it and see what gives. If anything. There's probably nothing there.'

He sighed. 'Okay. I'll talk to a few people and get back to you.'

Three days later, he was back.

'No big mystery in the end, but a lot of secret squirrels going on.'

'What do you mean?'

'So. Your man's a bit of a storyteller, it seems.'

'What's it all about?'

'This is all totally unofficial. He hasn't got cancer. He's got a girlfriend instead. A week with the missus and a week with the girlfriend. No-one is suspicious. He was one devious bugger.'

'Okay.' I thought about it.

'What will you tell the coroner?'

I thought again. 'Difficult. Probably that he drowned due to a rogue wave.'

'And the cancer?'

'Maybe I could say: "I could not find any evidence of cancer at autopsy." Something like that? It's technically true, after all.'

'Sounds good. And the family will say: "What a shame! There he was, cured of the cancer and he has to go and drown!" Those waves can be a serious bugger, though. Cheerio then.'

Sometimes society has to just get on with it. No point making heavy weather about things. There's more than enough of that out there at the best of times.

CHAPTER 17

The Privy Council and Beyond

Parliament Square in London has a pleasing symmetry. Dominating the Square are the Houses of Parliament and Big Ben standing on the east side. To the west side stands the Supreme Court, and Her Majesty's Privy Council, which for much of New Zealand's legal history, was the court of last resort for the United Kingdom and her former dominions and territories. To the right of the Supreme Court on the south side stands Westminster Cathedral and St Margaret's Church, which in turn face directly across the square to Whitehall, offices of the executive of the Civil Service.

Standing upright, between them all, and scattered across the lawns of the Square is a convocation of ten statues. Some stand proudly looking on with imperial disdain while others stand with attitudes of conspicuous humility. They are the statues of the good and the great, of those who have served their country and the countries of its former empire well: from Winston Churchill to Lord Palmerston, from Field Marshal Smuts to Nelson Mandela and Mahatma Gandhi.

There they stand as the guardians between the different organs of the state, as if to remind each of their duty to stand separate and apart — the Lords and the Commons to make the Law, the Courts opposite to interpret the Law, the Civil Service to enact the Law and finally the Church to cloak all with a suitable spirituality.

I climbed the stairs from the Westminster tube station to the Square, surrounded by civil servants hurrying to their jobs in the daily administration of government. I had made my way through the rush-hour bustle of early-morning London all the way from Shepherd's Bush. I was an hour and a half early, but I didn't want to be late for the first session of the Privy Council in hearing the appeal in the matter of R v *Lundy*.

London and the Privy Council was the last place I thought any evidence of mine would be heard, and nothing was going to stop me from hearing it given.

I sat on one of the old dark oak benches in the public gallery of the court and looked around. There was a smattering of public already there. I saw Detective Sergeant Ross Grantham. Our eyes made contact across the room and he nodded. A few journalists, identified by their recording equipment, were whispering to each other, looking around, no doubt trying to determine who was who. Who could give them a good angle for their stories, they seemed to be asking. I avoided making eye contact with them.

The Privy Council and Beyond

Between the public gallery and the Law Lords' benches were the seats and tables of the learned counsellors for the Crown as respondent, and for Mark Lundy, the appellant. Cameron Mander and Annabel Markham were seated on the right. Cameron was to present the case for the respondent. This was going to be a fight needing strength, endurance and clarity of thought. I was fully confident that Cameron was up to speed with the nuances of the case. David Hislop QC, sitting on the left, appeared for the appellent. Each principal lawyer had a retinue of scurrying acolytes carrying large cardboard boxes full of files, files and more files, all bursting with papers. The acolytes scratched amongst the papers like anxious mice, making sure everything was in place, ready to go when their senior crooked his or her finger.

What on earth can all this paper show? I wondered. The truth never changes. The case still seemed extraordinarily simple to me.

High on the eastern wall of the courtroom was a large window. The outside was smeared with the exhausted outpourings of the city. Inside, the glass was coated with a patina of sere dust. I wondered how old that dust was. These grimy layers admitted an indifferent, cold light, penetrating dimly from the downcast day.

Below the window was a clock, its long hand lurching from minute to minute. I would come to know that clock well, especially while watching the hands make their arthritic journey around its moon face.

Today, the clock was 20 minutes slow.

The Cause of Death

The Law Lords filed in, accompanied by the Chief Justice of New Zealand.

Lord Hope of Craigshead presided. To his right sat Dame Sian Elias, Chief Justice of New Zealand, and Lord Reed; to his left were Lord Kerr of Tonaghmore and Lord Hughes of Ombersly.

It was very impressive, I have to say. These were the doyens of law in the Her Majesty's realm; they were the finest legal minds in the United Kingdom and the dominions.

'My Lords, my Lady.' The Queen's Counsel for the appellant, David Hislop, was addressing the court. He covered an impressive range of topics, from computer viruses to petrol consumption, but I listened with particular interest whenever he raised the pathological arguments.

'I beg you to believe that the evidence that I am laying before you is fresh evidence. It is not merely a revisiting of evidence from the first trial in 2002. It is completely fresh evidence that has only recently come to light because of the efforts of an eminent scientist. I implore you not to think that we have traversed the world merely shopping for an expert, for anyone at all, just to find an opposing point of view. The evidence I shall lead is a significant departure and improvement upon what was heard previously in 2002. I respectfully put it to you that this case is an example of the critical reliance placed on "bad science" to secure a conviction, that very sort of conviction that Hammond J addressed in his opinion in the Queen and Wallace. On those grounds alone, we respectfully submit that an appeal should be granted.'

The Privy Council and Beyond

He looked up. The Justices were regarding him intently. Lord Hughes was making a note.

'My Lords, my Lady, although the identification of the brain tissue on the plaintiff's shirt is evidently the major and most serious issue that we bring before you to consider, that solemn matter is indeed not all,' Hislop continued. 'It was a significant component of the Crown's original evidence that Christine and Amber Lundy were murdered at precisely 7 p.m. This time, in turn, depended solely on the process of gastric emptying. We will be bringing before the court substantive and expert evidence that this position is erroneous and quite unsustainable. I would point out to the Court that Justice Ellis, in his summing up to the jury in Mark Lundy's first trial in 2002, made the point very clearly that for the prosecution to succeed, then the time of death of around 7 p.m. was essential. If, on the other hand, the jury was not satisfied that the evidence sustained this, or were left in reasonable doubt, then it would be fatal to the Crown's case.'

I nodded in admiration. He was a very impressive orator, clear, precise and very convincing. My assurance that the facts of the case were simple began to evaporate. This was going to be a tough argument to win.

'Furthermore, we say that it will be the appellant's case that in the original trial, counsel for the defence did not contest the truth or reliability of the brain tissue on the shirt and nor was there any meaningful challenge to the error of basing the time of death on gastric emptying. These issues have therefore never been rebutted in open court and that alone makes the original conviction unsafe.'

The Cause of Death

* * *

We heard all of the opening arguments and then broke for lunch. At the lunch break, I went down to the cafeteria and ordered a sandwich and a pot of tea. Ross Grantham joined me. I had seen him chatting to a couple earlier. He told me that the woman was Mark Lundy's sister. She and her husband had travelled over to London to offer their support. It was a long way to come and no doubt very expensive. I was impressed by their family loyalty and solidarity.

Ross told me that one of Mark's friends and supporters had told him he knew Mark was innocent.

'How could he know?' I asked.

'He said it was because he knew Mark well. He reckoned if I knew him as well, then I'd know Mark could never have carried out those murders. I told him that unfortunately I never knew him personally, so I don't have that luxury. All I have to go on is the evidence.'

* * *

The session went on and, as promised, it was all about the identification of the brain tissue on the shirt. How sound was the test? How valid was the evidence? Full and frank and robust presentations were delivered by both the Crown and the counsel for the appellant.

Most of it was familiar and was picking at old bones that had already been thoroughly gnawed in the original trial. A disproportionate amount of time was spent arguing about whether the original dab slide I had been shown was the same as, or different, from the revealing slides later made in Texas and if so, how did that change things. It was an irritating and irrelevant argument, and it could shed little light on the central question in the case: were Christine's brains on Mark's shirt or not?

To my mind, it was as if you had passed a barely legible roadside sign reading WELLINGTON 150 KILOMETRES and pointing in an aimless direction and then, some time later, you had actually arrived in the capital city and were driving up and down the streets. The sign had been like the dab slide, pointing the way to go. Rod Miller's brain preparations were like being in Wellington. Why on earth would you debate what the road sign looked like, or in what direction it was pointing, and whether it proved Wellington truly existed when you were actually in Wellington? Yet that was precisely what they were doing.

'But perhaps Counsel could help me here?' Lord Hughes said with his usual debonair politeness. 'As I understand it, we have two completely opposing scientific points of view. Surely you're not asking us to choose between one and the other? How on earth would we know which was correct?'

'My Lords, Ma'am.' Cameron, for the Crown, rose to his feet. 'Our experts are of the opinion that the scientific evidence proffered by the defence is in fact not scientific at all.'

'From where do you draw that conclusion, Mr Mander?' Lord Hughes looked at him intently.

'I draw your Lordship's attention to the affidavit presented by Professor Gown from the University of British Columbia.'

The Justices all leafed through their heavy volumes of documents and found the indicated place.

'Yes, yes,' said Lord Hughes a trifle tetchily. 'Please continue. I think I have the place.'

'My Lords, my Lady. We say here, and I quote, that this analysis is not science, it is not a scientific document, and it is merely intellectual gamesmanship,' Cameron said, and looked hopefully up at the Justices.

Lord Hughes laughed, his cheeks pink with mirth. 'That's not factual evidence, surely? That's merely vulgar abuse! It strikes me that what this issue cries out for is to put these differing experts from all around the world into one room and allow them to develop a consensus view, so that we may then know what to think of the matter.'

'Brilliant!' I thought. That suggestion was eminently sensible and probably should have happened many, many years ago. But of course, pragmatism and the law are at best nodding acquaintances.

So the long afternoon wore on.

Argument and counter-argument were advanced but they all led nowhere.

I could see that the pathology was going to be the weakest link and that was a surprise to me professionally.

I saw it like this. The Law Lords had been given two distinctly different arguments. The one from the Crown we all know very well because it never changed. The tissue on the shirt is brain. Because it is well preserved and had to be rapidly dried it must have landed there during the murder. Whoever was wearing the shirt is therefore the murderer.

Counsel for Lundy, on the other hand, were frustratingly single-minded. I thought they had a preconceived idea and they were sticking to it, a bit like a fundamentalist's religion. Their approach was simple: 'If it was brain tissue then it must have been decomposing for weeks by the time it was examined and so it cannot possibly have been preserved. There's therefore no point even look at it or discussing it, because there can't be anything there.'

This argument was barren. It didn't offer any scientifically credible alternative suggestion as to what it was we saw on the slides. It merely denied it could be brain tissue. The frustrating thing for me, a pathologist accustomed to finding fact, was that somewhere and some time the question would have to be faced if the truth were to be known.

I spoke briefly to Annabel. 'I don't really care how many eminent professors say our work was wrong. The truth never changes and I stand by it. But I do know one thing for certain. Only one of us can be right.'

It was a long and intense day. I couldn't see any way on earth the court could settle this controversy without a thoughtfully directed cross-examination of expert witnesses. But I had begun to see the lie of the land: only a retrial could offer that.

* * *

Gastric emptying. Is gastric emptying a marker in establishing the time of death?

There is an entire galaxy of problems associated with gastric emptying. There are so many unknowns that it is the last thing that pathologists like to introduce into any homicide inquiry. It's just too imprecise.

Originally, James Pang had estimated the time of Christine's and Amber's deaths as occurring within an hour after last eating. This was based on the fact that both mother and child both had stomachs full of recognisable, undigested food. As the McDonald's meal had been bought and presumably eaten at 6.45 p.m., that suggested a time of death of around seven o'clock.

David Hislop presented evidence from Professor Bernard Knight, a giant of forensic pathology who has written ten textbooks on the subject of gastric emptying, based on his experience of over 25,000 autopsies in his lifetime. Evidence from a man of that stature is nothing short of magisterial. He indicated that like most forensic pathologists and gastroenterologists, he believed timings based on gastric emptying to be unreliable to the point of worthlessness.

There is an interesting philosophical point in this debate. I have always wondered how any pathologist — even one of Professor Knight's stature — could actually get the quality of experience that would yield a true answer. In most cases, the pathologist has only a rough idea about when the people they are autopsying last ate. How, then, could pathologists of all people ever judge how quickly gastric emptying happens and how reliable a marker it is? After all, it is a dynamic process that only happens in the living. Yet here we were, basing opinions upon our experiences exclusively with the dead. Surely you would have to measure gastric emptying times in normal, healthy living people or else you would just be guessing? Lord Kelvin got it right. He said: 'If you can't measure it, then it is not science.'

Lord Kelvin would have approved of London-based Professor David Silk, who tests gastric emptying in the living, and has turned it into a measurable science. He gives people with normal digestion a meal that is balanced for carbohydrates, fats and proteins, all mixed with a radioactive marker and observes the digestive processes. He has a real-life knowledge of emptying time for normal people who have had a normal meal. And he says that in normal people, 90 per cent of the meal is still in the stomach after one hour and 60 percent after two hours. Only 10 per cent remains after three hours.

I often wonder how Professor Silk's evidence would have illuminated matters had he been called in this case.

* * *

The next morning, I sat in what had become my customary position, on the extreme left of the public gallery. I chose the farthest edge of the public gallery because it felt comfortably out of sight of the mainstream. It was hard enough listening to the lawyer for Lundy pounding and shredding my credibility and my evidence, without feeling I was under scrutiny as it happened. I could only grind my teeth in frustration and wait on events.

I found it frustrating, because there had been no opportunity to give a written answer to the appellant's second round of affidavits. The appellant had launched the first round, the Crown replied with the second, including mine, and these prompted the defence to prepare their final response. And that was it.

This was a pity, because there were some curious assertions in that unanswerable final salvo that cried out for robust cross-examination. One of these was that the brain tissue may have come from a sausage or a hamburger. While that may be possible in Britain, the home of mad cow disease, Kiwis would most certainly be shocked if there were any raw brain tissue in any of our hamburgers.

The other was a puzzling, unsupported claim that neither I nor Professor Peter Vanezis, Head of the Department of Forensic Medicine and Science at the University of Glasgow, were qualified to recognise brain tissue, as we weren't neuropathologists. No evidence was given for this bizarre claim, which would never be supported by any professional college. It was like saying you have to be a specialist dermatologist to recognise skin. Even medical students can recognise brain tissue at a glance.

We watched the Law Lords filing in. They too took their usual positions.

Lord Hope opened the proceedings. 'Could I ask counsel to limit their arguments to one hour each in this session?'

As politely as it was phrased, it was an order, not a request.

'Now that clock,' he pointed to the clock on the wall, 'is 20 minutes slow. I will need to call the court into recess at 12 o'clock for luncheon.'

His plea for brevity had no noticeable effect. The interminable arguments went on, both from the Crown and from the appellant, this expert and that expert, gastric fullness and gastric emptying ... Every now and then, the Law Lords would interject with some quibble or another.

'But surely, Mr Hislop,' Lord Hughes was asking, 'the Crown never had to prove precisely when Christine Lundy was murdered; the Crown only had to prove that Mr Lundy murdered her. In that sense is the time that it was committed relevant?'

'Whatever,' I thought wearily. It was predictably going nowhere.

* * *

The session that afternoon was fairly revealing, although I saw two reporters drowsing throughout. The tennis was on in a much more entertaining court. They longed to be there and so did I, but I was determined not to miss this.

We heard evidence of exactly why Mike Behrens QC ran the defence that he did in the original trial.

Lord Hope was speaking. 'Mr Behrens has retired, but has kindly sent a letter to the Registrar outlining the reasons for his conduct of the defence back in Palmerston North in 2002. I believe that it is pertinent to reveal these matters to the Board. I shall quote from his letter.'

He consulted the index to the files before him, turned and selected a volume, rearranged his glasses and began to read from the letter.

'— and I believed the Crown theory of the case, i.e. "the around seven p.m. murder" was nonsense. I believed that a far more realistic theory was that deaths had occurred after eleven p.m., perhaps in the early hours of the next day. I was aware that the Crown could be pushed into changing its theory. I was not to know that the Crown would not change to the after midnight theory.'

'It would seem then,' Lord Hope summarised, 'that Mr Behrens chose to defend based on the seven p.m. time and not to challenge the evidence about the stomach contents. He considered it to be the only time on which the defence had the potential to unhinge the Crown's case.'

'That is a reasonable stance,' commented Lord Kerr. 'But while it is true that before the trial, one could not have been certain that the prosecution might not switch to an alternative theory of the timing of the deaths, surely after the trial began, a change on such a vital issue was unfeasible?'

* * *

'I would like to move on in the interests of the shortness of time,' said Lord Hope, 'but first I will address the more narrow issue of the defence approach to the nature of the tissue on the shirt. It is clear that the prosecution had the shirt tissue examined by a Professor Vanezis, as well as by Dr Synec, a forensic neuropathologist. Those experts were of the view that brain tissue was present. Faced with this overwhelming consensus, it is not surprising that Mr Behrens conceded that the polo shirt was indeed stained with brain tissue. This meant that the defence focus was not on the nature of tissue, since that was agreed, but rather on how it got there. The possibilities of accidental or deliberate contamination were suggested as possible methods. While indeed it may not be surprising, that concession means that Professor Miller's evidence has never been formally rebutted in a court.'

I knew then it was over. There would have to be a retrial.

* * *

The Princess Victoria in Shepherd's Bush was once a gin palace but now was the favourite restaurant of our daughter Victoria and her husband, David. Elayne and I pushed through the door into the welcome warmth, glad to be out of the biting wind ripping down Uxbridge Road. Victoria and David were already there, a bottle of Bordeaux open, two half-full glasses testifying that they had been waiting a while.

We sat down and David poured us each a full glass of the Bordeaux.

'How is the trial going? Any interesting bits?' Victoria asked.

'Bad news for the Crown, I think. But it's been very interesting.'

'Why is it bad news?' Victoria's eyes were concerned. 'What's happened? I thought your evidence about the brain was very good. Everyone has always said it was very good.'

I explained what had happened.

'How is it possible that pathology experts can all have such completely different opinions?' asked David. 'I've always thought pathology was so scientific that you always got the right answers.'

That bothered me a lot, too. I had racked my brains — and I have done so since — for a logical reason but have found none. All I can say is that people can and do have odd ideas, and pathologists are certainly not immune. As G.G. Kelly put it, talking about ballistic evidence in murder cases: 'I soon learned the gun spoke eloquently, sincerely and truthfully; I have found that people sometimes fall a little short in this regard.'

People are, well, people, and we all hold a wide range of opinions. That is only to be expected and in one sense our ability to differ defines our humanity. But evidence is evidence too, and the truth never changes, no matter how much people wish it might.

Pathologists are certainly not always right and not even always unbiased. At times, their opinions can even be seriously aberrant. Indeed, one of the British defence pathologists in this hearing had conditions placed on their medical registration in 2016 after being found to have acted irresponsibly and beyond their expertise in a number of homicide cases, in that they showed a lack of objectivity, and sought to cherry-pick research that did not support their opinions. The court banned that pathologist from giving expert evidence in civil, family or criminal courts for three years.

Nevertheless, the appellant's experts had put forward their opinions and said why they thought they were right. I thought they were fundamentally wrong. I was really pleased the Law Lords had said my evidence was 'trenchantly asserted'. It sure was, and I did so because I knew it was right.

The Privy Council and Beyond

For all that meagre personal satisfaction, I was depressed by the outcome. I had genuinely expected the reason and logic of what we had put forward would prevail.

'What will happen now?' asked Victoria? 'Does this mean that Mark Lundy will be acquitted?'

'No, there'll be a retrial. We'll have to go through everything all over again and a new jury will decide.'

'That's terrible!' Victoria said. 'After all these years in jail and now to have another trial about the same stuff, all over again. Why not just let him go?'

'Well, it would be a much cheaper and easier option for us all,' I agreed. 'But I'm looking forward to a proper retrial for purely selfish reasons. I would like to know one way or another whether I was right or wrong. And right now I'm ravenous. I just hope to goodness there's no raw brain tissue in the food.'

* * *

It was late in the afternoon of the third day. I think everyone was exhausted. Counsel on both sides certainly looked weary. They had been on their feet for three days arguing, probing, and thinking under unrelenting intellectual fire from the Law Lords.

The Lords appeared to be exhausted, too. I had noticed that they were involved with several other cases at the same time. They had read and digested the tomes of files presented to them and it was clear that they followed the arguments and knew and understood them as well as anyone could.

The Cause of Death

I was tired. The benches were becoming harder the longer I sat upon them. They proved the truth of the old saying about similar seating in churches: the common factor between the divinity and those wooden benches was they both shaped your end.

But at last we were finished.

* * *

The judgement was eventually delivered by Lord Kerr. It was intellectual, comprehensive and unarguable.

'We have concluded that these matters may only properly be resolved by the triers of fact in a trial where a suitable and searching enquiry into all these areas of dispute may take place. The Board will therefore humbly advise Her Majesty that the appeal should be allowed, that the convictions should be quashed and that the appellant should stand trial again on charges of murder as soon as that can be conveniently arranged.'

So, there it was officially. *Regina* v *Lundy*. One-all. Round Three would be the decider.

And the clock on the wall was still 20 minutes slow as I left.

* * *

The retrial began in February 2015, some 18 months later.

The expert evidence again dominated the news. Again, the trial was everywhere — on the radio, the television, in the blogs, everywhere.

I didn't follow progress closely, but to my jaundiced ear, it all sounded suspiciously like the same evidence we had heard twice before.

But there were some significant differences.

First, the brain tissue evidence was finally decided. Two top international forensic neuropathology experts, Dr Daniel du Plessis for the Crown and Professor Colin Smith for the defence, collaborated and re-examined Rod Miller's work, repeated it and carried out more special stains.

The answer was unequivocal.

It was brain on the shirt, beyond any doubt whatsoever.

The defence now had to concede absolutely and without reservation that this was so.

I had always said both sides couldn't be right. I was relieved. The truth of the matter had been determined, and my pathologist's world was restored to its normal axis.

Better still, I heard the experts even managed to find evidence of brain tissue on the original dab slide using electron microscopy. And Daniel du Plessis confirmed that the whole argument about the lack of preservation was rubbish and a red herring. So we were right there too. Doubly vindicated!

The defence tried to resurrect the contamination argument, suggesting that maybe the brain came from a barbequed lamb chop. Of course, the fact that the only DNA that could be detected in the stain was Christine's and there was nothing of a lamb, was ignored. I burst out laughing when I heard that. This case seemed destined to go round in endless circles.

The Cause of Death

There was one completely new piece of evidence. Dr Laetitia Sijen from the Netherlands Forensic Institute found human messenger Ribonucleic acid (RNA) in the brain tissue. So that made it incontrovertible. It was brain, it was human, and the DNA testing said it came from Christine.

The Crown prosecution case for the time of the deaths was changed for the retrial. Death was now stated to be somewhere between when they bought McDonald's at six o'clock and when their bodies were discovered at 9.30 the next morning, but most probably occurred in the early hours of the morning.

That was now a pretty big window of opportunity. The defence now perhaps appreciated that Mike Behrens was extraordinarily astute in appreciating that only the original time of seven o'clock gave the defence any elbow room. Any later time was impossible to refute. The visit from the prostitute was no longer an alibi, and there was no need for that record-breaking drive from Wellington.

If the Crown's revision of the time of death was startling, the defence's gambit of using gastric emptying was breathtaking. They argued that the fact Amber's stomach was full of food meant that death in the early hours of the morning was impossible unless she had got up long after going to bed to eat her warmed-up McDonald's meal. Incredibly, they were now arguing *for* the seven o'clock slot. It seemed disingenuous to me, but the law is about advocacy, and that is how it works.

It has been pointed out by Mike White in a *North & South* article that the fries in a photo of Christine's stomach contents weren't shoestring fries, such as were served up by McDonald's. These were about one centimetre thick.

Pathologists develop an acute visual memory, and I can clearly remember that photo of the stomach contents taken so many years ago. Mike is correct. Shoestring fries are about two millimetres thick, while frozen oven fries from the supermarket are about seven millimetres thick.

Mike astutely suggested that Christine must have eaten another meal later in the night, and this is not so surprising, really, when you think about it. A McDonald's meal at six is not likely to have satisfied a woman who enjoyed food, and who by all accounts was a bit of a night owl. How everyone missed that in the first trial is a very good question.

It didn't really change anything, of course. So maybe the gastric emptying time of one hour was still right. Perhaps it occurred one hour after eating, but only after a much later meal, putting the early hours of the morning squarely into the equation. Who will ever know for sure now?

* * *

By now, the defence must have realised they weren't holding a very strong hand of cards. The brain on the shirt remained, as it always had been, the 'killer blow'. They needed something, anything, to counter the powerful run of evidence that had proved so conclusively that Christine's brains and her DNA were on the shirt.

They challenged Detective Senior Sergeant Nigel Hughes' security video of the original scene. A video of a relaxed scene at the Lundy home was shown to the court, with hairy male legs in jandals in the frame, indicating a man sitting on a couch in the house, apparently watching television. He seemed not to have a care in the world that he was sitting in the middle of murder investigation scene.

But it was wrong. Police videos taken at the Lundy's house at the time of the murders showed the house was well secured, protected by the well-known 'Police Emergency' tapes. Police officers and others investigating the scene meticulously kept to the steel stepping plates to prevent contaminating the scene. Definitely no-one sat and watched television while the enquiry was going on. The video that was shown was plainly shot at a different time, long after the event.

But the defence was grasping at straws. Christine's brains were unequivocally on Mark's shirt and everybody knew it, especially the jury.

The case limped on towards its inevitable conclusion.

Mark Lundy was again found guilty by a unanimous verdict of the jury at his retrial. He was sentenced to recommence his prison term of 17 years. He has never admitted to his crime. Another appeal will surely follow and his supporters remain staunchly behind him. No recent evidence presented in court has changed their minds. And nothing ever will. No level of proof can ever be high enough, and for them, there will never be any evidence that cannot be dismissed as falsification or conspiracy.

Afterword

Never send to know for whom the bell tolls: It tolls for thee.
— John Donne, *Meditation XVII*

Death, dying and the dead are inescapably part of us and our lives. One day, some time and in some place, we too will have our turn, for death is where it ends for all of us. When it happens, it becomes the task of the police, the coroners and the pathologists to ask the questions. It is they who have to make some sense of it all.

We as pathologists, we as a society, investigate death to try to discover answers, but to what end? What do those left behind actually want? Do they actually want to know? I think, quite often, what they want in their hearts is what the poor, demented husband in my first ever case wanted: the impossible, to turn the clock back and retrieve their loved one. I'm not immune to these feelings, and so often I wish

The Cause of Death

I could do just that for all the people I have written about in this book. But of course, none of us can.

All we can offer is to dissect the cold bodies of their loved ones, find the hard facts and display them in the bright light of reality so we can all know the how and the when and the why of their death. But that is a poor offering compared to what they want, which is for it never to have happened at all.

Why then do we bother to find out what happened if death is inevitable and if it is only a few relatives who really care?

These are important questions for us to consider. The foundations of our society are profoundly and solidly based on our science, knowledge and understanding. It is not logical to accept these foundations as a basic premise for everything, but then deny it to our dead and to our families when we die.

The stories of those who have died must be told, for they will enrich us all, as it is only in death that we find some meaning to our lives. By knowing and understanding death, so too may we also come to know and understand ourselves.

The Moving Finger writes; and having writ,
Moves on; nor all thy Piety nor Wit
Shall lure it back to cancel half a line,
Nor all thy Tears wash out a Word of it.
    — from *The Rubaiyat of Omar Khayyam*

ACKNOWLEDGEMENTS

I would like to thank the many families for the time they have taken to tell me their stories. It was my privilege to look after your loved ones and tell their story and I am grateful for your support. I owe a debt to the New Zealand Police who have always shown the highest integrity and professionalism in these investigations. The Coroners have been a fount of wisdom and compassion and I have learnt a great deal from their deliberations in court. Finally I salute my colleagues, those fine pathologists and mortuary assistants who are a great team of advocates for the dead and who do so much towards telling their final story.